Complementary
and Alternative
Veterinary
Medicine
Considered

There cannot be two kinds of medicine—conventional and alternative. There is only medicine that has been adequately tested and medicine that has not, medicine that works and medicine that may or may not work. Once a treatment has been tested rigorously, it no longer matters whether it was considered alternative at the outset. If it is found to be reasonably safe and effective, it will be accepted.

—Angell, M., Kassirer, J. P. Alternative medicine—The risks of untested and unregulated remedies. *N Engl J Med* 1998; 339: 839

There is no alternative medicine. There is only scientifically proven, evidence-based medicine supported by solid data or unproven medicine, for which scientific evidence is lacking. Whether a therapeutic practice is "Eastern" or "Western," is unconventional or mainstream, or involves mind-body techniques or molecular genetics is largely irrelevant except for historical purposes and cultural interest. As believers in science and evidence, we must focus on fundamental issues—namely, the patient, the target disease or condition, the proposed or practiced treatment, and the need for convincing data on safety and therapeutic efficacy.

—Fontanarosa, P. B., and Lundberg, G. D. Alternative medicine meets science. *JAMA* 1998; 280: 1618–19

There are no sects in science, no schools of truth. While facts of Nature are being studied out and until final certainty is attained, there may be legitimate and amicable differences of opinion in the scientific fold; but in ultimate truth there is an essential unity, and no contradictions are possible. The existence of conflicting sects and schools, for instance, of chemistry or astronomy or any objective science, is unthinkable; it is equally incongruous in medicine. The unenlightened public is unable to appreciate the solidarity of truth or to perceive the incongruity of conflicting divisions in medicine or other sciences.

—Nichols, J. B. *JAMA* 1913; 60: 332–37

Complementary
and Alternative
Veterinary
Medicine
Considered

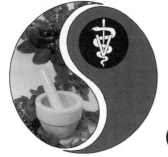

David W. Ramey
Bernard E. Rollin

Foreword by Franklin M. Loew

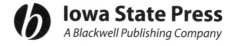

Iowa State Press
A Blackwell Publishing Company

David W. Ramey, DVM, is a 1983 graduate of Colorado State University. After completing an internship in equine medicine and surgery at Iowa State University, he entered private equine practice in southern California. Dr. Ramey has published numerous books and articles on equine health care, including the Concise Guide Series, and has lectured extensively. His interest in and research into "alternative" veterinary medicine led to his being selected as a member of the American Association of Equine Practitioners Task Force on "Therapeutic Options" and a member of the committee responsible for the current AVMA guidelines regarding the use of complementary and alternative veterinary medicine.

Bernard E. Rollin is University Distinguished Professor, professor of philosophy, professor of biomedical sciences, professor of animal sciences, and University Bioethicist at Colorado State University. He earned his BA from the City College of New York and his PhD from Columbia. He was a Fulbright Fellow at the University of Edinburgh. Rollin is the author of numerous books and papers dealing with animal ethics, animal consciousness, animal pain, and biotechnology. He has lectured over eight hundred times in eighteen countries. He is the founder of the field of veterinary medical ethics and is a principal architect of 1985 laws protecting laboratory animals.

© 2004 Iowa State Press
A Blackwell Publishing Company

Iowa State Press, 2121 State Avenue, Ames, Iowa 50014

| Orders: | 1-800-862-6657 | Fax: | 1-515-292-3348 |
| Office: | 1-515-292-0140 | Web site: | www.iowastatepress.com |

Printed on acid-free paper in the United States of America

Library of Congress Cataloging-in-Publication Data
Ramey, David W.
    Complementary and alternative veterinary medicine considered / David W. Ramey and
        Bernard E. Rollin—1st ed.
        p. cm.
Includes bibliographical references (p.   ).
    ISBN 0-8138-2616-0 (alk. paper)
    1. Alternative veterinary medicine. I. Rollin, Bernard E. II. Title.
SF 745.5.R36 2003
636.089'55—dc22   2003017359

The last digit is the print number: 9 8 7 6 5 4 3 2 1

To the memory of Franklin Loew (1939–2003), DVM, PhD, scientist, veterinarian, teacher, humanitarian, historian, dean of two veterinary schools, college president, polymath, entrepreneur, wit, animal advocate, and loyal friend. His influence in all of these areas has been incalculable and will endure.

Contents

Foreword

For 250 years, veterinary medicine and its scientific underpinning, veterinary science, have struggled to gain the confidence and respect of clients, fellow health scientists and practitioners, and the general public. And it has been accomplished by means of the scientific method and strict objectivity. To embrace unproven or even discredited "complementary and alternative" techniques surely is regressive both for patients and for veterinarians.

Veterinary medicine has always been open and sympathetic to new treatment and diagnostic modalities, but only when they have been proven in controlled studies. In 2002, Abraham Verghese wrote in the *New York Times* about cancer in humans, "I am not a crusader against alternative medicines or its practitioners. I am all for things that make us feel better and that don't hurt us. But I do wonder at the paradox of even the most rational of us being drawn to these bottles with pictures of ugly tubers and weedlike plants on them. Why do we become dreamy-eyed hearing the songs of the New Age pied pipers whose melodies interweave quantum physics and the workings of the colon in beautiful but completely fictional ways? Like revivalist preachers, they invite our faith, our willingness to search for magic in ancient, undecipherable Oriental practices (as opposed to the new, quite decipherable, Western practices). In return they offer nostrums, tonics, tapes, books, diets, retreats, mantras, votive candles and cruises; they bring color, fragrance and incense to an illness experience that otherwise plays out in black and white."

This book is a masterful accounting of the "how" and "why" this seems to be happening. It is candid and pulls no punches. The ethical issues surrounding the use of unproven therapies loom large, and the authors fully address these. This book comes at the right time and is as important a book to veterinary medicine as textbooks of surgery or medicine.

Franklin M. Loew, DVM, PhD
President, Becker College;
former dean of the Colleges of Veterinary
Medicine at Tufts and Cornell Universities;
Member, Institute of Medicine,
National Academy of Sciences

Acknowledgments

Our deepest appreciation goes to

Dave Rosenbaum, without whose enthusiasm and support this and other projects would not have been possible

Linda and Mike Rollin, for open dialogue and trenchant criticism

Bob Imrie, DVM, for his unflagging devotion to sorting out the truth

Hilary Brown, for her commitment to animals, language, and intellect

Trenton Boyd, librarian and historian, without whose generous help and support much of the research in this book could not have been done

Jeff Basford, MD, PhD, for always entertaining questions gracefully

Paul Buell, PhD, who never met a language he didn't like

Paul Unschuld, professor of Chinese medical history at the University of Munich, for his support, help, and encouragement

Jackson and Aidan, for the love and light that you bring to the world

Vic Stenger, PhD, who knows all about the stars (just ask Jackson)

Introduction

Now that I have spent 25 years teaching veterinary ethics and working closely with veterinarians in virtually every area of veterinary medicine, it seems appropriate to make some autobiographical comments, particularly in regard to my recent skeptical work on alternative medicine. I commonly hear the complaint that I am not entitled to be skeptical regarding non-evidence-based, nonmainstream medicine because my own work on ethics was not evidence based, and was, in 1976 when I started the field, certainly not mainstream. Thus I, of all people, should be open to the deviant and unaccepted, since I benefited from openness and receptivity to new views.

This may seem like a strong argument, but ultimately it is fallacious. Ethical issues clearly existed in veterinary medicine and in science despite the fact that the scientific community was ideologically disposed to deny their existence, justifying that denial with the well-known rubric that science was "value-free" and thus, *a fortiori*, did not make ethical judgments. Thus, scientific ideology largely grew out of the attempt to expunge what is not verifiable and testable from science; ethical judgments are not verifiable, therefore, they were not considered to be part of science.

But the key point is that the ethical judgments were *there*, whether they were acknowledged or not! For example, every veterinary practitioner must ultimately make an implicit (if not explicit) commitment to whether he or she has primary moral obligation to the animal or to the owner; without such a commitment, the veterinarian could not make rational treatment decisions. The fact that such judgments were not previously consciously examined or even acknowledged did not stop them from being operative.

Similarly, every animal researcher has had to implicitly make the judgment that the knowledge gained from an invasive experiment was of greater value than the suffering in the animal it engendered. Thus, when I pioneered in calling attention to ethical issues in veterinary medicine, I was simply illuminating what had been ignored. I was not creating something *ex nihilo*. And in calling attention to neglected ethical issues, the social status of veterinary medicine was being strengthened, not eroded.

Is this analogous to being open to "alternative medicine"? In a trivial sense, it is. No advocate of science, including the authors of this book, suggests that it is impossible that new therapies may arise from implausible bases. We are quite willing to be convinced that other cultures, even so-called primitive cultures, might have arrived at promising therapeutic modalities—it may even be likely. However, this situation is not analogous to the ethics case. It is neither ethical nor scientific to claim that alternative modalities work *prior* to satisfying the canons of evidence that science and medicine have set up as justifying such claims. Advocating application of therapies that are antithetical to science is not like calling attention to ignored ethical issues; it is more like making a claim that there are deep supernatural issues in veterinary medicine, and demanding that they be considered. And insofar as veterinary medicine is chartered by society to be science based, not adhering to scientific canons weakens veterinary medicine, rather than strengthens it.

Thus, however open-minded I may strive to be, I am under no obligation to accept as therapeutic any modality that has not been tested by the criteria that scientific medicine uses to accept or reject mainstream therapies. On the other hand, I welcome and encourage the scientific testing of new modalities as well as any mainstream modalities that have been accepted without testing—the requirement of testing holds just as strongly here as it does in alternative medicine. As anyone trained in scientific methodology knows, it won't do to say "I saw it work"— with no proof of causation, we don't know that we didn't simply see this treatment followed by this phenomenon,, or that we aren't operating by wishful thinking, the Rosenthal effect, or any number of other biases. That is why double-blind randomized clinical trials serve as a "gold standard" for proof in science!

Other criticisms I have faced are equally ill founded. For example, one colleague chided me for proliferating animal suffering in demanding evidential bases for treatment. I pointed out that relevant evidence could first of all be garnered via clinical trials, without deliberately hurting animals or making them sick. In addition, I pointed out that using unproven therapies could also cause animal suffering. For example, many years ago I witnessed a disturbing "wet lab" involving surgery done on a rabbit with acupuncture. The animal was heavily sedated, restrained with leather straps, yet it still struggled and vocalized. The "true believers," however, saw what they wanted to see—"successful" surgical anesthesia. Additional suffering could occur if a therapy doesn't work, or if, by receiving an ineffective therapy, an animal is prevented from getting something that does work.

Another criticism I have received is equally troubling. "You," I have been told, "have directed many criticisms at science, from its denial of ethics to many other components of its unexamined ideological presuppositions. Yet here you seem to uncritically accept it."

Once again this criticism is ill founded. Unfortunately, too many people in society have polarized into proscience and antiscience. What veterinary medicine must try to do is to discard what is indefensible and hold on to what is valuable. This just makes sense. In my writings, I have pointed out that science has often been tainted with bias, corruption, favoritism, old-boyism, and so on. The exclusion of women from much heart research earlier in the twentieth century, the funding of AIDS research over breast cancer research, the protection of established theories (e.g., stress as a cause of ulcers), the powerful hegemony of paradigms (e.g., Freudianism in psychiatry earlier this century, replaced by biopsychiatry), the influence of economics and politics on such hegemony, the publish or perish system, all taint science and impair its alleged objectivity and tarnish the ideal of science as an objective path to empirical truth. But, in the end, science has built into it self-correcting mechanisms. Their effectiveness may vary, but they are there and will, we can hope, invariably become operative. No other modality for learning about the world contains such a self-correctional mechanism.

That I criticize science in some areas does not mean that I cannot view it as the best approach we have for gaining knowledge of the world. To my knowledge, no other method contains within itself the machinery for rejecting false conclusions, however slowly and haltingly it may work. Even Newton's authority could not save absolute space and time from Einstein's devastating critique; medicine eventually did establish that *Helicobacter pylori* causes ulcers, in spite of initial criticisms; and experiments that allegedly demonstrated cold fusion were ultimately shown to be flawed.

Looking at alternative medicine—or rather, the veterinary community's reactions to it—has led me to a disturbing conclusion reinforcing what I have learned in 25 years of teaching nascent veterinarians: our teaching and training are seriously deficient in the area of critical thinking. We are so busy making sure that students have memorized and can spit back the relevant facts that we do little to assure that they know how to use them and logically manipulate them. As an example, one of my colleagues at CSU, in fact a supporter of alternative medicine, invited me to address his class in complementary and alternative medicine. "Challenge them [the students]," he said to me. "Make them think." I began by asking them to think about what science can and cannot do. For example, I suggested that science cannot confirm or deny the claims of those practitioners who claim to be able to speak with the souls of sick and dead animals, allegedly taking advice from these souls regarding electing humane euthanasia. "Surely," I confidently affirmed, "science cannot test claims about communications with souls." "Why not?" far too many students chimed in. "You are putting illegitimate limits on science." In other words, they could not grasp the difference between an empirically testable question or claim and one that could not be empirically tested! This in turn displays an appalling lack of conceptual sophistication among those supposed to be scientifically trained.

To paraphrase Kant, learning facts without the ability to reason about them is empty, even as learning reason in a factual vacuum is blind. Not only in veterinary medicine, but also in all disciplinary education, we are doing more training than educating, and we are failing to assure that students can reason and logically manipulate the material they learn. Even more disturbing is the fact that a significant number of students of mine who are candidates in the sciences were favorably disposed toward using unproven alternative medicine, despite an almost total lack of empirical evidence in its favor in terms of efficacy or safety. This in turn evidences that even in the case of these students whom we are training as scientists, there has been a failure to grasp the rudimentary principles of scientific reasoning.

If veterinary educators confront this appalling lack of critical thinking ability in our graduates, then the debate over alternative medicine will have strengthened our ability to produce graduates who can reason in both veterinary medicine and veterinary science. But if we do not heed these disturbing signs, veterinary medicine may well relegate itself to a world of medical anarchy, where no approach to knowledge or treatment has pride of place, because there are not objective standards for proof and truth, and "anything goes."

I was fortunate enough to begin my career in veterinary medicine by teaching with Dr. Harry Gorman, arguably one of the greatest veterinarians of the twentieth century, inventor of the artificial hip joint, supervisor of the aerospace program's use of animals, founding member of the American College of Laboratory Animal Medicine, president of the AVMA. In addition, Dr. Gorman was instrumental in conceptualizing what he, two others, and I turned into federal law, assuring the well-being of laboratory animals. He was what he liked to call a "closet philosopher," possessed of sound common sense and Humean skepticism always aimed at pomposity, nonsense, and obfuscation. I learned enormous amounts from him. One thing he constantly stressed was that veterinary medicine had found its way from obscurity and lack of academic status to a highly respected position in medicine by ever-increasingly hitching its wagon to scientific inquiry, and accepting nothing in the absence of evidence. "Above all else," he admonished me, "make sure that we never lose our way by failing to observe the principles of science, common sense, and common decency." I dedicate this work to his memory and to the spirit of that admonition, though I doubt he could have guessed how readily some of his colleagues would abandon that which moved veterinary—and human—medicine into high social credibility. For this reason, I gratefully acknowledge Dave Ramey's drawing me into this fray when he phoned me and said, "You helped teach me how to reason, now I need your help in defending it."

Bernard E. Rollin

I am a practicing veterinarian who specializes in the care and treatment of horses, with 20 years of experience gained from almost daily work "in the trenches." I have seen my clinical work glorified and vilified, and I've seen promising therapies come and go. In the crucible of clinical medicine, where no one has all of the answers, the only constant is the parade of options available to make things better for the horse. You work hard and do the best you can.

The learning curve in the practice of veterinary medicine is initially steep. When one enters the field, new facts and ideas come at a frenetic pace, defying even the most committed efforts to absorb them. However, after several years of study and experience, the slope of the curve tends toward the horizontal, and the realization that we are relatively poorly armed in the fight against disease and injury takes hold. And it was at that time, perhaps 12 years ago, that I became drawn to alternative veterinary medicine.

I recall being fascinated with the ideas that other cultures had wisdom that had eluded those of us unfortunate enough to be limited to Western ways. I became interested in learning what other approaches to the care and treatment of patients involved. At the core, I was hopeful that I would learn new and better ways to help the horses for which I care. I attended lectures and seminars on such things as acupuncture and chiropractic, and I was duly impressed by the enthusiasm of the presenters and encouraged by the promise of the new and the strange. I even went so far as to request application for acupuncture certification—but something always nagged at me.

That something was the lack of intellectual sophistication in the presentations that I had heard. It was weird. In the course of my education, both pre- and postgraduate, I had been to countless lectures. I had even published research of my own. I was comfortable in the scientific debate; I relished the opportunity to dig deep into questions and look at the trail of ideas that led up to current thought; I reveled in the stimulating debates. But in my initial forays into alternative medicine, I was dismayed by what I found. Rather than critical analysis, I found naïve acceptance; rather than a respect for scientific education and rigorous methods of analysis, I found cults of personality and messianic zeal. Rather than evidence of effectiveness, I found testimonials. Not being one who is swayed by authority, I began to look into the field on my own. And, in the time-honored tradition of science, I began to publish what I found.

At about the same time, I began to see the influx of nonsensical ideas into my own geographical area. For a short time, many show horses were being shod with a pad on one fore foot and the diagonal hind. Why? Their legs were uneven. How did we know? "Ask the chiropractor." Did such pads make a difference? Not that I could determine. After a year or so, horses were no longer shod in that fashion. I haven't seen it done in years. Perhaps I'm lucky enough to now be taking care of a group of horses with even legs. More likely, they never were uneven at all. Nonetheless, my practice career has seen a nonstop parade of magnets and lasers and acupuncturists and massage therapists and psychics, and it doesn't look like it's ever going to slow down. But they've all gone away—or at least the initial furor died down. Charades can't last forever. But a new game, with new players, comes along every day.

The veterinary profession needs to get off this merry-go-round. The history of medicine is instructive. We have thousands of years of ghastly and/or ineffective medicine. Thousands of years of treatments that providers thought worked, and that in fact were killing and maiming the animals: bleeding, burning, purging, cupping. Thousands of years of doing things that maimed and killed—or doing things that did nothing at all—and doing them over and over and over and over and over again. Never stopping once to do rigorous tests to see whether they were actually safe and effective. Tormenting a new generation of animals with the same things that tormented their sires and dams, and their sires and dams—and describing them as time-honored treatments. Sprinkled among the lethal treatments may have been a few that worked, or at least did not cause overt harm. But most of those—like putting ice on an ankle sprain—have already shown their worth. We need to move on.

Say you're driving from point A to point B. There could be any number of routes to get there. You might choose the route that takes you by the park, or the one that takes you by the lake, or several other alternatives. The thing that all routes have in common is that you're going to get where you want to go.

Say, however, that there's another route that will take you on a long drive but you'll never end up at point B. I suppose one could consider that route an alternative to the other routes, but why would you want to take it? In fact, it's not really an alternative at all, if you consider the term *alternative* to imply another way of achieving your goal (point B). Taking such a route would be a complete waste of time.

That's the beef with the alternatives to established therapies that get discussed in medicine. People should not be restricted in how they reach their destination—it's just that if they're going to go on a trip, they should be able to have a pretty good assurance that they're going to get where they want to go. To extend the analogy further, people embarking on such an alternative route may even enjoy the ride, stopping for gas, buying food, the lovely conversation, and so on, but what's the real point of the trip if they're going to end up somewhere out in the woods? And what about those who sell the alternative route takers on the wonders of their "new" directions—are they practicing a "new paradigm" of cartography?

So here's the next question: is it acceptable for a professional to just do anything under the guise of good intentions? Or do they have an obligation to show that we're actually doing something helpful for the animals for which we care? If they do have such an obligation, then clearly, they must separate safe treatments from unsafe, and effective from ineffective. Clearly, they then need to use some method to do so. And, clearly, they've got that method in place and most veterinarians would seem to agree that they should use it. And, to a large extent, they have, and alternatives to scientific medical practice have consistently been found wanting.

So what's the allure of alternative medicine? It's the appeal of the healer; the call of the hero; the desire to help, even when all hope is fading. It's the fear of death and disease, the realization that there's no cure for every ill, the unwillingness to say, "I can't do any more." It's innumerable systems for innumerable conditions with formulas and theories and even the best of intentions. But it is not scientific medicine. And it has been science, after all, that is the only thing that allows veterinarians to rise above all others who claim to be able to help treat animals.

Thus, there is this book. This book is the other side of the coin. It promotes no particular therapy. It is not against alternative medicine. Rather, it is a lengthy exposition on various aspects of the whole, diverse field. It is based in research, not anecdote. It also carries a strong bias—a bias for effective therapies, for science as the best way to flesh out empirical claims, and for truth. Would that the entire profession shared such a bias. All would be better for it.

David W. Ramey

Complementary
and Alternative
Veterinary
Medicine
Considered

1

The Braid of the Alternative Medicine Movement

Various unrelated and diverse therapies are euphemistically described as "holistic," "alternative," "complementary," or "integrative"; in veterinary medicine, the popular acronym is CAVM, for complementary and alternative veterinary medicine (with so many names, some, as per the suggestion of medical historian James Whorton, might even call it vernacular medicine). Many interesting questions can be raised regarding these therapies, including, "What are the reasons for their apparent popularity?" and "Why now?"

The questions are intriguing, but the answers, while easy to speculate, are difficult to substantiate. Yet the temptation to answer is overwhelming. Undoubtedly, no one single factor can explain the whole phenomenon. Certainly the factors vary in importance and in their temporal appearance. Some even become self-perpetuating or combine with their antecedents to become apparently new again.

We gratefully acknowledge the assistance and contribution of Wallace Sampson, M.D. Dr. Sampson is board certified in internal medicine and is a Fellow of the American College of Physicians. He is a Clinical Professor of Medicine at Stanford University, where for 20 years he has taught the analysis of dubious medical claims. He is editor-in-chief of the Scientific Review of Alternative Medicine.

Some material for this chapter is adapted from Sampson, W. The braid of the "alternative" medicine movement. *Sci Rev Alt Med* 1998; 2(2): 4–11, with permission, Prometheus Books, Amherst, NY.

PREDISPOSING AND ANTECEDENT SYSTEMS

Many predisposing psychological and political influences account for the rise of "alternative" medicine. In addition, the traditions of various cultures may hold clues as to why alternative medical approaches have proliferated. For example, in Germany, *Naturphilosophie* was a widely supported, although much criticized, general view of nature, popular at the beginning of the nineteenth century. It started by seeing divine patterns being repeated through the world, both inorganic and organic, and ended with something close to pantheism, identifying people with a larger creator. Add a tint of Samuel Hahnemann's homeopathy, which prescribed infinite dilutions of substances to affect "vital forces," Rudolf Steiner's anthroposophical medicine, which purported to reintegrate humans with the world of the spirit, and a few mystical legends, and one may discover a German tradition of "alternative" thinking. In Britain, the tolerance of the unique, eccentric, and bizarre appears to be something of a source of national pride. In Asia, the sense of tradition is also strong, and spirituality and cosmology have been partnered there with all phases of life since records have been kept.

In North America, such influences may include the traditional mistrust of authority that characterized the earliest settlers, including government, politicians, elitists, and professionals. Historically, North Americans adopted a mélange of folkways from European countries, and combined them through the eighteenth and nineteenth centuries into a new brand. For example, North American herbalism evolved from a blending of Native American herbalism and European household medicine, through the vitalist underpinnings, codification, and popularization of the practices by Samuel Thomson in the nineteenth century. W. K. Kellogg developed a process of manufacturing a breakfast cereal for sanatorium patients that revolutionized American breakfasts and popularized concepts of nutrition as the key to health. The cereal maker C. W. Post, who made his first cereal product in a sanatorium; the clergyman Sylvester Graham, a rip-roaring advocate of temperance, vegetarianism, and the graham cracker; and Mary Baker Eddy, the founder of Christian Science, all interpreted and recombined vitalistic concepts. These in turn passed through people such as D. D. Palmer (the founder of chiropractic) and Jack La Lanne, in human medicine to such people as Andrew Weil and Larry Dossey, and in veterinary medicine to such people as Allen Schoen and Susan Wynn. Deregulation, the lack of governmental oversight, economic considerations, and do-it-yourself medicine, perpetuated by the rise of the internet and the resulting easy exchange of anecdotes and information, appear to play a part in the more recent wave of interest in alternative approaches to medicine.

People separate slowly from folk methods. They stick to the common consciousness. In addition, people may be reluctant to accept new ideas, or ones that are not easily understood. It is much easier to reflect and repeat the quaint ideas and irritating habits with which people are familiar. For example, the idea that toxins build up in the human colon was one of Kellogg's basic premises (he called it "putrefaction"). Such revelations were proclaimed to the unawakened public. Efforts to remove those toxins resulted in the feared, torturous enema, in fact, something of a punishment for having gotten ill, but one that was to be eagerly solicited by those with ill-founded concerns. "Colonics" are still in vogue in some venues today. Indeed, "There is no branch of knowledge in which error is so wide-spread and deep-seated, or looseness and superficiality of thought so prevalent, or theorizing, amateurism, faddism and mysticism so general, as in the field of medicine."[1]

Long-established customs die hard. They appeal to those who want to explore the past for overlooked nuggets of wisdom, to those who long for a simpler time, or to those who hope to find answers to unanswerable questions in mysteries. Historians and psychologists note that these emotional-spiritual undercurrents of need are strong determinants of behavior. On the other hand, technical, professional, scientific medicine is only about a hundred years old. There is no long-established tradition. It may seem foreign and inaccessible. As such, those with alternative approaches can easily reject scientific medicine.

But there is certainly more. For example, one may point to a growing concern, particularly in the industrialized countries, of the risks and dangers associated with an indiscriminate application of modern sciences and technology to shape human life and exploit the natural environment. Disasters from Bhopal in India to Seveso in Italy, from Three Mile Island in the United States to the pollution of the Rhine River by the Swiss chemical industry in Germany, have almost certainly contributed to a widespread hesitation among Western populations to trust in chemistry, physics, and modern technology as the sole means of constant progress and perpetual improvement of quality of life.

In fact, with the improvement of relations between the former Soviet bloc and the West, environmental concerns appear to have largely supplanted the prospects of a nuclear war as the dominant existential fear in industrialized nations of the West. As a result, such fields as chemistry and technology, which previously appeared to have only positive connotations, began to lose their attractiveness, despite the fact that almost any aspect of daily life was unthinkable without chemistry and technology. Regular reports about the negative effects of chemistry on the cleanliness of air, soil, and water, on animal life and the safety of food, and hence on the body and its health, caused chemistry to be seen in a different light, and provoked fears that extended to modern medicine.

The same general process of change can be seen in attitudes toward technology. The impact of technology on daily life, once celebrated in world exhibitions as the solution to the millennia-old problems of humanity, now came to have a pale aftertaste for a certain section of the population. According to that section, technology is felt to destroy nature and also to destroy relationships between human beings. The picture of the railroad and freeway is no longer associated principally with communication between distant regions; it is equated with the carving up of stretches of land once intact.

This increasing aversion to the impact of chemical science and technology on human life has repercussions in various arenas of Western civilization. Environmentalists have raised their voices, and so-called Green parties have been able to express the fears of their voters in national parliaments. Nuclear power plants have come under attack, and a general "back to nature" attitude has affected food habits, clothing, and the construction of houses.

Health care has been no exception. Health care is the response of humans to the most serious threat to their existence or to the existence of their animals, that is, illness and the risk of early death. Modern veterinary medicine uses modern chemistry and technology, much as in human medicine, and hence it has come under suspicion as polluting and harming the individual animal's body, in the same way that chemistry and technology pollute and are claimed to destroy the environment. Such fears and suspicions may help account for the wider trend that provides numerous types of traditional and alternative health care with a faithful clientele.

Still, whether an undercurrent or a propelling force (a case could be made for either), the essence of all these threads seems to lead to a loss of standards for thought and action and a disregard for intellectual discipline. Combined with a celebration of individualism, the cultism associated with followers of strong personalities, and their messianic zeal, "alternative" approaches challenge the rigor and routine that characterize scientific medicine.

CULTURAL RELATIVISM

Cultural relativism was born in the early twentieth century in the innocence of academic fairness and objectivity. Its intent was to omit prejudice and emotion when investigating other cultures. Previously, the trend had been to describe other cultures with xenophobic, supercilious descriptions that even extended to American subcultures. Observers of such cultures typically used pejorative terms such as quaint, backward, primitive, pagan, and savage to describe them. Relativism raised cultural anthropology from biased emotionality of supercultures and superraces to realistic, judgment-free, academically productive understandings. It allowed an appreciation for the healthy diversity of human cultural evolution.

But cultural relativism became inappropriately applied. As applied to medicine, cultural relativism is a blunt instrument. As such, relativism has been applied to medical systems as if they merely reflect cultural differences instead of being approaches that were more or less useful for increasing health and longevity. Judgment-free descriptions of health systems have replaced evaluations of their objective value to health. In relativistic schemes, the number of days of illness, numbers and sizes of epidemics, mortality rates, life spans, cure rates, misery, and pain are all ignored. Instead of valuing a medical system by how well it works, the measure of a medical system became how well it helps the culture's functioning and cohesiveness. This disconnect persists despite scientific data about modern biomedicine's obvious objective benefits.

Under a relativistic scheme, worthless and/or harmful traditional remedies are rationalized as being just different, alternative, traditional, unorthodox. Acupuncture, for example, may be rationalized by saying "if it has worked for three thousand years, there must be something to it" (even if the historical record doesn't support such a history of longevity or widespread use). Furthermore, "worked" is never quantitatively defined; neither an objective endpoint nor a treated condition is ever described. Conversely, questions as to why, if it worked so well, there is still such controversy about it, or why such a successful tradition might have been discarded, even temporarily, are overlooked. In addition, such arguments are selective; the test-of-time argument could be said for tiger parts or rhinoceros horn used for male potency. And broader perspectives may be ignored, for example, the ramifications of the decimation of wild animal species in order to reap the imagined effects of their parts does not seem to enter many perceived benefit equations.

Culturally based medical practices may also offer solace to people's fears. For example, the modern philosophical evolution of "traditional" Chinese medicine achieves some success because it is contrasted with the fears that may beset some people in the West. Until the 1960s, a feeling prevailed that in the long run things could only become better. An occasional war or economic crisis may have caused hardship, but the long-term perspective was one of confidence. The vast majority of Western people were confident that life eventually could only improve.

This confidence has been severely shaken over the past several decades. The long-term developments of such things as the purported global climate change, an increase in natural catastrophes, the loss of fertile soil, the increasing competition for water, and the growth of world population have, for some, replaced confidence with despair. Whereas previously the prospects for improvement of the human condition were good, for many the future now appears bleak, with no solution in sight. It is here where such foreign concepts as the Chinese "yin-yang" and the "five-elements" doctrines became attractive to some.

The contrasts between scientific and nonscientific medicine are dramatic. Take Chinese medicine. The yin-yang and the five-elements doctrines are based on cyclical thinking. Both promise the return to an origin. The five-elements doctrine has an additional inbuilt mechanism promising solutions for crisis situations. If wood is too strong and endangers soil, the son of soil, that is, metal, emerges and cuts wood until it is no longer able to penetrate soil. That is to say, each force leading to crisis provokes the emergence of counterforces controlling this force and, hence, leads to the end of the crisis. Since Western science may not be trusted to provide answers and to offer solutions to such crises (real or imagined), cyclical yin-yang and five-elements doctrines may appear as viable alternatives. In fact, many Westerners have lost their faith not only in modern Western science but also in traditional European, that is, Christian religion. One might even say that for some of these people these alternative doctrines have become what may be called a secular religion.

It is the task of religion to answer the most fundamental questions on human existence. Humans wish to know their place in the universe. They wish to know what they must do to survive and what they must avoid lest they perish. Conventional religions respond to these questions by outlining a moral code established by one or more numinous beings. A secular religion answers these questions by pointing out the morality required by natural laws. Western science does not offer such a morality; Chinese traditional methods (and other such philosophy-based systems) do. Through a belief in the yin-yang and five-elements doctrines, people may find answers to their most pertinent questions. Through these doctrines they learn how to survive and how to safeguard their own existence and that of their fellow beings. The yin-yang and five-elements doctrines offer definitions of righteous behavior and of sin. Finally, and importantly, they offer what Westerners appear to have longed for most, that is, confidence—a confidence that some cannot find in the naturalistic approach of science. Uncertainty may be one of the most difficult things for the human mind to tolerate.

Cultural relativism also results in a peculiar blindness to folkways' untoward consequences in favor of nonjudgmental descriptions. For example, at the meeting of the American Association for the Advancement of Science in 1979, sociologists convened a conference on laetrile, a fraudulent cancer remedy. The criminal backgrounds of promoters and the biochemical implausibility of laetrile were de-emphasized; no physician, biochemist, or pharmacologist was invited to speak. A sociologist commented on another presenter's critique, "[Prof.] Rich's [critical] paper is the most difficult to treat because of the bias I perceive. . . . His view is as valid as mine, so I present these thoughts as an alternative view to consider. . . . Any analysis of laetrile must carry some bias; even neutrality is a bias. . . . [A]ny bias will do as well as another. . . . He should consider the degree to which his perceptions and conclusions depend on his particular bias rather than on 'objective fact.' "[2]

Thus, through the nonjudgmental, relativist eyes of the medical sociologist, even fraudulent medical schemes and cults are viewed as merely cultural differences. As such, educated opinions become biases, whether they describe violation of laws of physics, chemistry, and pharmacology, or laws of the land. As such perspectives proliferate, people grow farther from, rather than closer to, the truth.

POSTMODERNISM

The derivative of cultural and philosophical relativism is the postmodern view exemplified by Michel Foucault, Jacques Derrida, Sandra Harding, Paul Feyerabend, and other philosophers of science. These individuals view science and knowledge as merely social constructions, relative to the individual's view or to the society in which the knowledge is created, as opposed to its being a method to search for immutable truths. Postmodern values significantly predict attitudes to and actual use of alternative medicine in humans;[3] there is every reason to suspect that a similar finding would be made regarding the use of CAVM.

Some versions of postmodernism deny the existence of an outside world or universe (or disease or treatment) that can be measured objectively and upon which one can take reasoned action. In a parallel manner, some alternative medical systems—such as acupuncture, homeopathy, or chiropractic—may rely on the manipulation of invisible or unmeasurable forces, and practitioners of those systems are not dismayed by the fact that those forces cannot be shown to exist. The result of such positions is the dissolution of measurement and a world devoid of facts. Under such constructs, all judgments become subjective.

Much of the liberal arts and social-science academic community was devoted to the postmodern viewpoint for the last several decades of the twentieth century. Two generations of students have been educated in it, going on to take places in the legal community as attorneys and judges, in politics as officeholders, and in the media as reporters, editors, and producers. Administrators of granting agencies—both public and private—grounded in relativistic/constructivist principles, determine where and to whom research grants go.

Postmodern editors, and even staffs of professional journals, may be affected by the "niceness" straitjacket and the relentless search to ferret out bias. In the same vein, courses in CAM (complementary and alternative medicine) are taught in most medical schools without critique, evaluation of validity, or even historical accuracy. Judgments are to be eschewed, options embraced.

MONEY

There has always been a fringe of healers, doctor wanna-bes, willing to dispense information for a price, or just for the satisfaction of appearing to be real scientists and medical professionals. These individuals often supply methods rejected by scientific biomedicine. Others make and sell products with debatable or no effects, some of which may even compete with effective pharmaceuticals. The cumulative efforts of these individuals have succeeded in convincing a minority of the public of the power of supplements, antioxidants, athletic fuel, brain food, and special diets (to name a few). Bookstore sales on health, nutrition, and medicine are high, and magazine racks overflow. The competition for space is fierce. There has always been good grazing along the fringes of medicine.

But now wanna-bes are taking shark bites out of medicine's flesh. Techniques of sales, propaganda, legal maneuvering, and political contribution have reached significant levels. For example, the dietary supplement industry significantly influenced the representatives who wrote the Dietary Supplement Health and Education Act of 1994. That bill liberalized marketing of supplements and removed the Food and Drug Administration's preemptive control over unsafe products. As a result, companies now market products without proof of effectiveness and flood the marketplace with unstandardized, sometimes toxic, herbs and supplements. These products may even be embraced by professionals, who may choose to increase their bottom line rather than educate consumers about the untested and unproven nature of this endless stream of products.

At the same time, organized chiropractic and other occupational guilds repeatedly seek increased scope of practice, claiming to be able to diagnose and treat as physicians or veterinarians and lobbying for increased access to patient populations. Their political contributions may even help retool legislatures.

Private foundations and wealthy individuals fund many "alternative" activities and may even be their largest source of funding. Funds from private foundations have been spent on television programs, published studies on the use of alternative medicine, medical school departments and courses, postgraduate physician education courses, and research projects. Private funds helped establish the Argus Institute & Shipley Natural Healing Center at Colorado State University. Endowments for the pursuits of alternative approaches to human medicine are in the hundreds of millions of dollars, with annual funding exceeding the one hundred million dollars per year of the Federal Office of Alternative Medicine. Private foundations are the products of wealthy entrepreneurs with private ideologies they would like to see adopted by society. Financially strapped universities and medical schools accept these funds under conditions not acceptable a decade ago. For example, a few years ago, Yale University declined a contribution from a conservative donor on ideological grounds, and was hailed by the academic community. With a few exceptions, such circumspection is not apparent today.

PROPAGANDA AND LANGUAGE DISTORTION

Language is the supreme weapon in the battle to influence opinions. Its insidious appropriation and manipulation by the alternative medical world, both denotative and connotative, is worthy of challenge. Language is the one element that everyone claims equal rights to, regardless of intentions or competence. Attempts to demand its responsible use are typically met with defensive responses. Given that there is a smorgasbord of beliefs and positions even within one defined camp, it becomes a Herculean task to try to enforce definitions. Still, when it comes to alternative medicine, strict definitions must be demanded—but are often avoided—and the more fundamental the level, the better. Simple minds comprise fierce armies, but they are called to action by clever minds that know how to manipulate language at the earliest opportunity. Language is a battle in which alternative medicine proponents have already gained significant ground.

Proponents of unusual medical practices have put language to good use, and have succeeded in manipulating the public mind. For example, the words *holistic, alternative, complementary, unconventional,* and *unorthodox* are invented euphemisms. They are benign terms covering a vast array of practices—most of them unproved, dubious, disproved, absurd, and fraudulent. Any politician knows one must find an enemy, even a straw one, to win elections. Thus, instead of providing good evidence of effectiveness, advocates of the bogus cancer therapy laetrile demeaned ethical cancer medicine by inventing the phrase, "slash, burn, and poison." It worked and it stuck, and it echoes today.

In a strange twist of the alternative braid, constructivist sociologist-historians of medicine in an alternative medicine journal have turned the tables on such analyses of language distortion and have accused rationalist scientists' use of realistic terms like *quackery, misrepresentation,* and *fraud* of being merely prejudicial and biased.[4] They call for more neutral terms to describe absurd methods such as homeopathy. The intertwined strings of relativism and propaganda complement each other in the braid.

MISREPRESENTATION OF RESEARCH RESULTS

Most of the alleged positive reports pertaining to alternative medicine show serious defects. These include selected endpoints, analysis of aggregated data as if they were homogeneous, extraordinarily large confidence intervals with minimal significance, selected reporting of differences in recorded curves, miscalculations and misrecording of data, omissions of control and other objective data, and combining different disease categories into meta-analyses. Why peer reviewers miss such errors or allow publication of papers with such obvious errors is unexplainable.

However, once they appear, such errors become self-perpetuating. For example, a meta-analysis appearing in the British medical journal *The Lancet* in the fall of 1997 recorded the results of homeopathy studies at face value, despite the paper's faults. The meta-analysis is now a reference for the claim that homeopathy cannot be entirely explained by placebo action, even though several subsequent and more rigorous analyses demonstrated that paper's serious flaws (see chapter 7). Nonetheless, once inaccuracies in alternative medicine are reported as fact in medical literature, they are there for posterity.

BAD DOCTORING

Although there are certainly no data to support such a contention, it is not unreasonable to question the judgment of physicians or veterinarians who hold closely to ideologically driven methods that lack validity. The public usually has little sense for the quality of physicians, and there is little evidence that publication of lists of "best doctors" alters patient behavior. Most of us want medical practitioners to be top quality, but apparently there are other criteria besides objective outcomes by which quality may be judged. A practitioner's putative open-mindedness or genial bedside manner should be no substitute for the rigorous and relentless evaluation of results and ideas.

THE PRESS

The press is a major vector for the spread of alternative medicine. Typically, newspaper stories are uncritical—even inaccurate—and supported by warm-hearted tales of improvement from happy consumers. Unfortunately, these stories often fail to include any information about the lack of clinical data supporting—or refuting—such practices. Often, skeptical or scientific viewpoints are a mere afterthought. And, of course, there's rarely, if ever, any follow-up. Newspapers don't generally concern themselves about such things as how patients do in the long term. These are facts most medical professionals must have in order to give truly informed consent, although they may be less important to journalists, who may only provide isolated vignettes.

While outrageous claims may be highlighted, more sobering statistics may be harder to find. Still, examples of critical reporting can be found. For example, the July 3, 1998, *San Jose Mercury News* bore a small *Washington Post* article about rural China's 70 percent infestation rate by various parasites, most commonly worms, resulting in malnutrition, decreased intelligence, and general weakening of the workforce. However, the article was buried on page DD5, whereas the previous week's acupuncture article was on page 1B, complete with half-page photo. (This kind of editorial treatment seems typical.) And, of course, there is the unanswered question "Where are acupuncture and moxibustion when they are most needed?" Worm infestations apparently do not respond to alternative approaches. In fact, the failure of traditional Chinese medicine in China and its low usage there is a testimonial to modern biomedicine's success.

Unfortunately, the press is also often scammed. For example, in the August 16, 1998, issue of *Parade* magazine, there appeared an article about the marvels of acupuncture, including a smiling woman undergoing chest surgery with only ear acupuncture for anesthesia. The photo appeared to be a fake, as did the story—chest surgery without intubation and heart bypass or cooling is unimaginable.

In their own defense, reporters may say, "My duty is to inform, to present both sides, and let the (readers, patients, etc.) make up their own minds." To some, this seems to be simply a rationalization, perhaps to avoid having to do the hard work that characterizes the best reporting. However, judging from the numerous uncritical presentations that simply repeat common knowledge and uncontrolled anecdotes, hard work is not common when it comes to reporting about the world of alternative medicine.

POWER POLITICS

Traditionally, a distinguishing feature of those who promote unusual medical practices has been this: if they cannot prove their claims scientifically, they use the popular press and lobby for special privilege in legislatures. In human medicine, 27 states legalized laetrile as a cancer therapy in the 1970s and 1980s in spite of no evidence that it was an effective treatment. Twelve states have passed "access to medical treatment" (AMT) bills. These allow any licensed practitioner to practice any method within the legal scope of practice—proved or not—on any patient, provided informed consent is obtained. Chiropractors have legal standing to correct "subluxations" in almost every state. This authority was granted in spite of the fact that subluxations, as defined by chiropractors, have not been shown to exist. Pressure groups from the alternative medical community support these policies and contribute funds toward their passage. Political pressures, not public need or scientific validity, have been behind the rise of chiropractic, acupuncture, and other methods.

GULLIBILITY, MISPERCEPTIONS, AND THE WILL TO BELIEVE

Much is written about the human traits mentioned above, maybe too much to describe usefully here. But the fact is that people tend to want to believe, and tend not to want to take the time and effort to explore for deeper truths.

Alternative medicine may provide emotionally satisfying explanations for complex medical problems. These explanations may be at once mysterious, formulaic, and applied across the board and, as such, be readily embraced. Unfortunately, they are also generally wrong.

Books, such as *How We Know What Isn't So* by Thomas Gilovich, *The Psychology of Anomalous Experience* by Graham Reed, *How to Think about Weird Things* by Theodore Schick, Jr., and Lewis Vaughn brilliantly expound on concepts such as gullibility of the will to believe. Any number of papers on belief perseverance by Lee Ross and others, "Cults in Our Midst" by Margaret Singer, "The Psychology of Transcendence" by Andrew Neher, "Deception and Self-Deception" by Richard Wiseman, "Memory" and "Eyewitness Testimony" by Elizabeth Loftus, and chapters by James Alcock and Barry Beyerstein in *The Encyclopedia of the Paranormal* add to the knowledge base. Martin Gardner and James Randi give entertaining explorations of other oddities such as faith healers.[5,6] It behooves a reasoned observer to seek out informed sources.

CONCLUSION

The braid of the alternative movement is complex and strong and will always lurk in our backgrounds, even if all misery and disease were to be conquered. For now it grows into the interstices of scientific and ethical medicine's weaknesses and is fertilized by imagined faults. The movement has advanced socially and politically, although it has barely made a ripple in the pond of science.

One might look at the alternative medical movement as a swinging pendulum. Perhaps the pendulum is starting the swing back. For example, according to Prof. Edzard Ernst of Exeter University, the fascination with alternative medicine may have already peaked in the United Kingdom, and classes suffer from chronic underbooking.[7] In 2002, the European Community prepared to introduce legislation to provide a consistent level of consumer protection for people taking extra minerals and vitamins.[8] More recently, large corporations, such as Wal-Mart, as well as several states that make up the United States of America (Vermont, California, Indiana, Michigan, Minnesota, New Hampshire, New Jersey, Ohio, and Texas), have announced that they will either not reimburse patients for or dramatically cut back on patient reimbursements for chiropractic services.[9,10]

However, medical history shows that changes in the fundamental conceptualization of health and illness have never been based on clinical success of a new system of health care ideas. All over the world, ideas have been developed and accepted and applied in clinical practice, even when there were no clinical effects that could have justified this new practice. It is the ideas themselves that are convincing and attractive; proof of clinical success (or lack thereof) has always come later.

Still, much can be learned from alternative medicine's existence and social successes. Misinterpretation of events and the formation of beliefs can be studied, and the understanding of social movements can be increased. Medical historians must search for the reasons why a new system of health care ideas appears attractive. It is not as simple as it may appear at first glance. No single cause may be named as sufficient to provide a new health care system of ideas with plausibility. Perhaps it will be possible to tease out small kernels of benefits—even if only psychological—in some methods. Nevertheless, the challenge facing medical professionals—indeed, facing all of human society— is to increase their abilities to observe, measure, record, analyze, and reason, and not allow the holes in their reality-sieve to widen until they have lost their grip on them.

2

Historical Aspects of Some CAVM Therapies

Unlike most therapies used in veterinary medicine, CAVM (complementary and alternative veterinary medicine) appeals to longevity as a form of proof of efficacy. While certain therapies in scientific medicine may indeed have stood the test of time, the passage of time is neither the *only* means by which such therapies have been tested, nor the rationale by which such therapies are supported. Unfortunately, in the case of CAVM therapies, much of what has occurred over the passage of time has been misrepresented. Furthermore, the passage of time is not itself a particularly persuasive test. For example, astrology has persisted for thousands of years in spite of the fact that there is not one shred of objective evidence to support its myriad and diverse claims.

Nevertheless, most of what is described as "alternative" veterinary medicine might reasonably be regarded as well grounded in the traditions of many cultures. Paradoxically, while CAVM advocates describe what most mainstream veterinarians practice as "traditional" medicine, in fact, it is CAVM methods that often stem from traditional practices and belief systems that predate science. Throughout history, people and presumably their animals have always suffered from premature death, disease, and injury. It is likely that for just as long, people have tried to intervene in ameliorating those conditions. For example, therapeutic phlebotomy (bleeding) has one of the longest and best documented records in the annals of medical therapeutics. However, it has only been one hundred or so years since it was generally discarded, and the practice is still employed in some indigenous cultures in an effort to "drain out sickness."[1]

There is also nothing new about the current enthusiasm for unconventional therapies. For example, an 1850s source noted "Homeopaths, hydropaths, eclectics, botanics, chrono-thermalists, clairvoyants, natural bone-setters, mesmerists, galvanic doctors, astrologic doctors, magnetic doctors, uriscopic doctors, blowpipe doctors . . . etc., etc., etc." as just some of the many options that were available for medical consumers of that time.[2] Comparable levels of support for therapies that buck the medical mainstream have been the norm for most of the past several centuries. Furthermore, the characteristics that distinguish unconventional practices and their practitioners—claiming to be side by side with nature, reliance on personal experience over scientific data, and viewing patients as unique individuals—have also been remarkably consistent. Finally, the analysis of alternative claims by scientific practitioners has also been remarkably consistent, with most such claims failing to stand up to scientific scrutiny.[3]

It is true that today people and animals in modern societies are healthier, suffer less, and live longer than their ancestors. Most of the increase in longevity has occurred within the past century, side by side with the development of modern medicine. Those who rave about the long history of various traditions and procedures among various civilizations ignore the fact that those traditions and procedures were not responsible for any measurable improvement in overall health.

Still, even in light of the current appeal of some traditional or "alternative" therapies, there is no excuse to distort the historical record in an effort to legitimize them. Indeed, because some advocates of such therapies suggest that the mere fact that they have been in existence for a long time means that they must work, an accurate recounting of history is critical for an overall evaluation. Mystical and ancient healing practices are certainly worthy of study, both for their historical interest and for the possibility that they may ultimately yield some useful interventions. However, when viewed in light of historical accuracy, many alternative practices lose some of their luster, and, perhaps, some of their appeal.

ACUPUNCTURE AND TRADITIONAL CHINESE MEDICINE

The most recent wave of interest in Chinese medical practices dates to 1972, when U.S. President Richard Nixon visited the People's Republic of China, ending nearly a quarter century of China's isolation from the Unit-

---

"Acupuncture and Traditional Chinese Medicine" was written with the assistance of Paul Buell, PhD.

ed States. Among other revelations, traditional Chinese healing practices were presented to the Western media as the quintessential Chinese medicine (and were even employed on one member) and as a system equal, if not superior, to Western medicine. However, with the introduction of Chinese healing practices to the West and the great curiosity about them, some rather widespread and fundamental misunderstandings of what traditional Chinese medicine is and was appear to have gained widespread credence.

Indeed, a tendency can be recognized in the writings by Western authors on Chinese medicine to associate Western medicine with all the disadvantages of modern science and technology, and to identify Chinese medicine as a perfect alternative, although historically there is little justification for such clear-cut antagonism. In addition, several conceptual ideals supposedly unmet by Western medicine have been attributed to Chinese medicine—for example, the assertion that Chinese medicine is more holistic than Western medicine—although history does not lend itself to the support of such attributions. It is of interest to note, however, that one of the early best-sellers on Chinese medicine, the book *The Web That Has No Weaver* by Ted J. Kaptchuk (St. Martin's Press, New York, 1983) made just these false claims and has influenced the perception of Chinese medicine among tens of thousands of readers.

Another basic misconception is that Chinese medicine, as currently practiced in the West as so-called traditional Chinese medicine (TCM), is a reflection of the traditional medicine that is most commonly practiced in China, and, furthermore, that the medicine that is practiced in China is a true reflection of ancient practice. Neither premise is correct. In fact, the Chinese medicine of the tenth century is different from that of the first century, which is different from that of the nineteenth century.[4] The Chinese medicine that is being practiced in the United States and Europe is not the same as the healing systems being practiced in East Asia. Furthermore, the systems being practiced in either locale today are far removed from the practice of Chinese medicine prior to the twentieth century. Indeed, "what is very much now an 'alternative' Chinese medicine is only a minimal vestige of ideas and practices . . . extracted from a highly impressive variety of medical thought, and supplemented with modern elements of Western rationality."[5] Chinese medicine, in the sense of a homogeneous system of ideas and therapeutic practices, did not exist prior to its promotion as such in the twentieth century and does not exist today.

Instead, the entirety of beliefs and knowledge of preventive and curative strategies developed and applied until the middle of the twentieth century may be reasonably described as "Chinese traditional health care." It is also possible to speak of the entirety of medical theories and practices thought of, propagated, and applied in the previous two millennia as "Chinese traditional medicine." However, this is in contrast with so-called traditional Chinese medicine (TCM), which is a digest from traditions developed between the 1950s and the early 1970s. The distinction between traditional Chinese medicine and Chinese traditional medicine is not merely semantic. The adaptation of Chinese medicine promoted in China as *zhongyi* since the mid-1970s is, in fact, not an accurate reflection of the tradition of Chinese medicine measured from ancient times to the present.

In any case, the transformation of Chinese traditional medicine into TCM from the 1950s to 1970s did much to bring Chinese medicine closer to modern rationality. As previously noted, TCM is an abridged version of the vast heritage of Chinese traditional health care beliefs and practices. Most elements of Chinese traditional medicine that directly contradict modern science and rationality have been omitted from the many publications on *zhongyi* published in the People's Republic of China since the mid-1970s. Hence, Westerners returning from China in the late 1970s and 1980s took home a "gift," which they considered to represent two millennia of Chinese medicine while in fact it was a streamlined body of concepts adapted to modern rationality. It is this streamlined body of knowledge, then, which was once more modified in the West to meet the expectations of Western audiences.

The notion that there is a vast gulf between traditional Chinese and traditional Western medical practices is also completely without foundation. Indeed, the theoretical bases for some traditional Chinese medical practices are very much like those expounded by contemporaneous European physicians: for example, the Chinese had *qi* and the Greeks had *pneuma*, and early European missionaries at least assumed that the two words were synonymous.[6] In addition, there was a well-described tradition of drug and herb-based therapies, the prescriptions for which were, as today, simply based on recognition of the problem and subsequent selection of the desired substance,[7] which had absolutely nothing to do with mystical concepts and which mirrored medical therapeutics in contemporaneous cultures. It is only in modern times, with the development of science-based medicine in the West, and the subsequent discarding of metaphysical approaches to medicine, that Chinese (Eastern) and Western practices have been brought into opposition.

The earliest traditions of Chinese medicine (Shang dynasty, seventeenth to eleventh century B.C.) were tied to beliefs in ancestors, who were capable of endangering or even destroying human life. Healing practices were directed at restoring not only the living but also the dead. Later, magical, demonological, or supernatural beliefs pushed ancestral medicine into the background, and unseen demons became the cause of all disease (such beliefs still persist in some parts of the Chinese population). Demons residing in the body caused such things as swellings, and insertion of such things as needles or lancets could be employed in an effort to kill or expel them.

The real formative period of Chinese medical traditions was during the Han dynasty (roughly second century B.C. to second century A.D.). During the Han, the Chinese intellectual elite first attempted to reduce the phenomena of the world to a limited number of causes and effects, and Chinese health care took a decisive turn.[8] Natural laws, instead of magic or demonology, laid down in such doctrines as "yin-yang" and "five elements" were used to explain health and disease, and to legitimate preventive and therapeutic strategies. This was the beginning of a medical science in China, although the term *science* should be thought of only in its broadest sense. By comparison to what came before, it was more rational, but Han medical theorists certainly did not reject all earlier notions of demonological and ancestral influences on human health. These influences continued to exist in a rational Chinese medicine much as magic of various kinds continued to exist, for example, within a "rational" Greek and Roman veterinary tradition (e.g., Apsyrtus and his translators).[9] Nevertheless, the founders of Han Chinese medical science placed their primary trust in natural laws, presumably working independently of time, space, and human or metaphysical persons. From that time forward, a Chinese medical philosophy coexisted and interacted with ancient versions of health care that continued the belief in spirits and ancestors as responsible for human health and disease.

This new way of thinking made it possible for Han Chinese to try to understand natural processes as well as to influence them. Thus, theories involving such ideas as yin and yang, *qi*, and five phases evolved and were used in an effort to explain normal and pathological body functions. However, such theories were neither ubiquitous, generally accepted, nor consistent. For example, one school of Chinese thought subdivided the two categories of yin and yang into four yin and yang subcategories whereas a second school proposed three subcategories for both. Both of these schools of thought, though contradictory, appear to have agreed in their rejection of the five phases doctrine that is so important to other Chinese theories.[10] The Chinese apparently never made any attempt to resolve such contradictions. As might be expected, this has resulted in many factions within the domain of traditional Chinese medicine (TCM) and even more within the realm of what later became acupuncture.

Two distinct traditions of medical literature became apparent in post-Han China. Pharmaceutical and prescription literature were developed and applied without reference to what has been described as theories of "systematic correspondence,"* developed in terms of arcane, and often contradictory, interactions of yin, yang, *qi*, and the five elements. By contrast, an acupuncture literature that developed elaborated those notions. In this literature, as theories of systematic correspondence became more and more dominant, anatomy and physiology tended to become less significant and little more than symbol. As a result, "in the history of Chinese medicine, rather than progressing from a reasonable, although incomplete, knowledge of the body to a more detailed one by systematic dissection, the medical writers go in the opposite direction, under the sway of the cosmologists, to a less accurate picture."[11]

Although efforts to unite the two traditions were made, particularly in the twelfth–fifteenth centuries, those efforts were never entirely successful. Indeed, Chinese medicine "took the form of a stream flowing into an increasing number of separate and sometimes criss-crossing river beds" and became "nothing more than a complex labyrinth, in which those thinkers seeking solutions to medical questions wandered aimlessly in all directions, lacking any orientation, and unable to find a feasible way out."[12] Indeed, since no objective criteria could be used to show that one system was superior to another, escape from the tangled web of Chinese philosophies was impossible.

Western medicine was introduced into China in the nineteenth century; the twentieth century "has brought the further development of Chinese medicine within the confines of its traditional theoretical foundations to a complete halt." Science-based medicine has largely supplanted traditional practices in China and most recent estimates are that only about 15–20 percent of people in China currently employ traditional therapies.[13]

---

*Systematic correspondences followed a system of "magic correspondences" in history. In magic correspondences, the Chinese attempted to order the world in terms of an elaborate sympathetic magic. For example, the ancient Chinese saw a walnut and envisioned an open brain. They *do* look alike. Hence people in antiquity assumed that they must be related. To extend the correspondence, it could also be postulated that if one were to eat walnuts, the brain would be strengthened. Magic correspondence has many facets; however, the main point is that the world was seen as a conglomerate of countless separate (i.e., mutually unrelated) pairs of correspondences. In early Han times came the great conceptual jump: all world phenomena, tangible or not, were related through a system of correspondences. In this view, all phenomena could be influenced by changes elsewhere in the system. The body and its functions were part of the systematic correspondences, too. The medicine of systematic correspondences was, as a consequence, built on this type of ordering in the world. All emotions, all functions, all morphological entities are considered part of the more encompassing universe of systematic correspondences; the organism in all its functions and morphological units is tied to the seasons, to the surrounding physical environment, and so on. To neglect this system may result in disease; for example, if in winter one behaves as one should in summer, bad things might happen.

Nevertheless, TCM is now advertised in the West as a "natural" medicine. In fact, although the label "natural" is widely used in descriptions of Chinese healing, there is every justification to deny TCM the status of natural medicine. This label offers a false impression of security that the body will not be polluted with chemicals if a physician uses traditional Chinese pharmaceutical substances, although this was never a rationale for Chinese use of medicinal plants. Similarly, although acupuncture may appear to be safe because it does not rely on chemistry and introduces no chemical substances into the human body, such considerations were not made when it was first employed.

Certainly, Chinese medicine is not without its appeal to some. For example, the Chinese diagnostic process of inspection, listening and smelling, inquiry, and pulse taking is laborious and time-consuming and is carried out by the practitioner through direct contact with a patient. Such diagnosis requires no technological apparatus; it aims to evaluate the suffering of the individual, not to compare the patient with standard values, any deviation from which is *a priori* considered morbid. While low in scientific content, such interactions may be high in psychological value for the patient (or its owner).

Another important factor for the success of acupuncture and TCM has been the notion of *qi*. Chinese medicine, as interpreted by Western writers, at least promises to solve the "energy" problem within the individual's own body. By grossly disregarding the historical meaning of the concept of *qi*, by rendering *qi* as energy, and by explaining disease in terms of "energetic disturbances," the newly invented Chinese medicine has gained plausibility. However, this plausibility arises out of conceptual adaptation to Western fears, not out of the historical reality of Chinese thinking.

A further conceptual adaptation to the concerns of a segment of the population in Western industrialized nations enhances the attractiveness of Chinese medicine and contributes to its success. Metaphors of killing, defense, and attack, which have become prevalent since the nineteenth century with the development of bacteriology, and more recently in the realm of popular descriptions of immunology in modern Western medicine, have been taken for granted in China since ancient times. Despite these facts, this brand of figurative use of language does not appear in the version of Chinese medicine propagated in the West. Modern TCM practitioners may assert that their therapies are gentle and natural; historical ones certainly did not.

Anyone afflicted by disease, seeking rest and harmony, finds it hard to come to terms with the fact that modern drugs are engaged in a belligerent struggle to destroy the enemy in the organism. Accordingly, the general public may be aware of the side effects of drastic chemotherapy from the war against cancer and may be anxious to avoid them. In contrast to reports from the battlefield of modern immunology, the modern theory of TCM freed of its historical martial metaphors gives the impression that it can lead patients back to the harmony of the great whole. Modern—but not historical—TCM theory offers solace whereas modern medicine offers only the uncertainty of a murderous battle (although many of the substances used in Chinese herbal medicine are, in fact, highly toxic and can kill if used incorrectly or to excess).

In any case, Chinese medicine as currently propagated in the West is a mirror image of neither Chinese traditional medicine nor traditional Chinese medicine. The reinterpretation of *qi* as energy and the elimination of martial metaphors have created a new, Westernized appearance of Chinese medicine that is increasingly distant from its historical past.

THE HISTORY OF ACUPUNCTURE

Acupuncture is not synonymous with traditional Chinese medicine (TCM), and TCM is itself not a homogeneous treatment approach. In spite of this fact, of all of the historical traditions of Chinese medicine, acupuncture appears to be a primary subject of the most recent wave of curiosity in the West. The chronology of acupuncture in human therapy is fairly well established, albeit along a somewhat rough and uneven timeline.

Neither archaeological nor historical evidence has been discovered that suggests acupuncture was practiced in China (in humans) prior to the mid–second century B.C. The earliest archaeological findings, from the 1970s, were four gold and five silver needles, discovered in the tomb of Han dynasty prince Liu Sheng (?–113 B.C.) in Hebei Province. Since these artifacts were found in association with other therapeutic instruments, they may have been employed in therapeutic "needling" of some sort.[14] The precise nature of this needling is unclear and it may not have been used for purposes that we think of today as acupuncture. (For example, according to the Chinese classic medical text *Huang Di neijing*, needles were also used to remove "water" from joints or to lance abscesses.)

The written record of acupuncture history is somewhat clearer. The earliest Chinese medical texts known today, a total of 14 medical texts written on silk and wood, were discovered in 1973 at the Mawangdui graves, sealed in 168 B.C.[15] The Mawangdui documents appear to provide a comprehensive picture of Chinese medicine as it existed during the third and early second centuries B.C., but among numerous therapeutic interventions, acupuncture is never mentioned.

The earliest literary reference to any kind of therapeutic needling (*zhen*) is found in a historical, rather than a medical, text, the *Shiji* [*Records of the Historian*] of Sima Qian, written circa 90 B.C. The *Shiji* mentions one instance of needling in the texts but that needling was not associated with a system of insertion points or with the fundamental system of conduits (described in later centuries) whose *qi* flow might be influenced by needling. Indeed, the story of resuscitating a dead prince with a needle placed in the back of his head is hardly a component of later acupuncture and may, in fact, merely reflect lancing of a boil or abscess. Interestingly, Jivaka, the Indian protophysician and the personal physician of the Buddha, also performed surgeries right in the center of the head, and much earlier,[16] if we may believe the Indian tradition.

It was left for the *Huang Di neijing*† to introduce the practice and theoretical underpinnings of what clearly became human acupuncture in the historical sense (i.e., the manipulation of *qi* vapors flowing in vessels or conduits by means of needling). The book, which comprises three distinct redactions, is made up from textual pieces by various authors writing in various times. Although it is not clear when individual pieces were written or included in the larger textual tradition,[17] the main content of the book dates from later centuries and the earliest surviving editions date to between the fifth and eighth centuries A.D.[18] Most of the texts available today went through final revision in the eleventh century. The *Huang Di neijing* introduced the idea that the body contained functional centers ("depots" and "palaces") connected by a series of primary and secondary conduits that allowed for influences (*qi*) to pass within the body and to enter from without.‡ Interestingly, the text largely ignores specific skin points at which needles can be inserted.

Nonetheless, the concept of invisible, vaporlike agents that are responsible for maintaining life and health is not uniquely Chinese. Indeed, the concept of a vital air or spirit is one of the main concepts of ancient medicine of virtually every culture. For example, the Greek physicians Praxagoras and Erasistratus, among others, hypothesized that arteries conducted the vital force *pneuma* and not blood.[19] This and other similarities have led to speculation that the information presented in the *Huang Di neijing* may simply be an adaptation of Greek medicine, and, in light of the interactions that occurred between China and the West in Han times, such speculation is not unreasonable.

---

†The title *Huang Di neijing* has been the subject of numerous English translations. The text, which is actually three separate books, can be translated in several ways. Some confusion about the title appears to stem from a mistranslation by Dr. Ilza Veith, who, in her translation of the book, suggested that the title be translated as "The Yellow Emperor's Classic of Internal Medicine." However, the title simply means the "Inner Classic of Huang Di." Huang Di is the name of the mythological Yellow Emperor, originally a god of the Yellow Springs of the underworld, thus his color. He is also sometimes referred to as the Yellow Thearch (Thearch = god-ruler). The "inner" (Chinese *nei*) means an inner or esoteric tradition transmitted from master to student (as opposed to *wai*, an "outer" tradition for public consumption). The Chinese word *jing* means "canon" or "classic." Accordingly, any translation referring to this text as being related to internal medicine is entirely wrong.

‡The older parts of the *Huang Di neijing* are influenced by instructions to treat illness by phlebotomy (bloodletting). It has been theorized that bloodletting eventually developed into acupuncture, and the focus shifted from removing visible blood to regulating invisible *qi*.

Doubts about the efficacy of acupuncture therapy appear early. Repeated statements saying that if one does not believe in acupuncture, one should not use it, appear in Han dynasty writings.[20] Subsequently, for unknown reasons, acupuncture lost much of its appeal by the middle of the second millennium. By at least 1757, the "loss of acupuncture tradition" was lamented and it was noted that the acupuncture points, channels, and practices in use at the time were very different from those described in the ancient texts.[21]

Eventually the Chinese and other Eastern societies took steps to try to eliminate the practice altogether. In an effort to modernize medicine, the Chinese government attempted to ban acupuncture for the first of several times in 1822, and the Japanese officially prohibited the practice in 1876.[22] By the 1911 Revolution, acupuncture was no longer a subject for examination in the Chinese Imperial Medical Academy.[23]

By contrast, during the Great Leap Forward of the 1950s and the Cultural Revolution of the 1960s, Chairman Mao Zedong promoted acupuncture and traditional medical techniques as pragmatic solutions to providing health care to a vast population that was terribly undersupplied with doctors,[24] and as a superior alternative to decadent imperialist practices. Although Mao apparently eschewed such therapies for his own personal health,[25] acupuncture and traditional herbal therapies provided Chinese political leaders an expedient and face-saving alternative to the only other health care option available to the masses: no health care at all. Although the subsequent promotion and revival of interest in various Chinese medical traditions have been an economic boon for China, there is no evidence that such a revival has resulted in improved health for the Chinese citizens.[26,27] Certainly, Chinese medical traditions provided no obvious benefit to the Chinese when they were the only treatments available; it appears that life expectancy in China and India was probably around 25 years in the nineteenth century.[28] As a result, Western medicine is in high demand in China. Curiously, the revived interest in such practices in the West is concurrent with the apparent waning of such interest in the East.

ACUPUNCTURE IN THE WEST

Westerners first became generally aware of Chinese medicine in the sixteenth century at the time of the first direct maritime contacts, although it is mentioned as early as the thirteenth in the travelogue of William of Rubruck.[29] In the sixteenth century, acupuncture reached Europe in the form of a few stray manuals now held by the Escorial in Madrid, Spain, upon the return of Jesuit priests from the Chinese Imperial Court, and the United States somewhat later. It has since been rejected, forgotten, and rediscovered again in at least four major waves, including the current one. For a time, acupuncture became fairly well established in parts of Europe, particularly in France and Germany (concurrent with Chinese attempts to ban the practice). Several prominent French physicians advocated acupuncture in the eighteenth and nineteenth centuries, but other, equally prominent doctors were not impressed, accusing proponents of resurrecting an absurd doctrine from well-deserved oblivion.[30] Nineteenth-century England also saw a brief period of popularity for acupuncture. However, by 1829, the editor of the *Medico-Chirugical Review* was able to write, "A little while ago the town rang with 'acupuncture,' everybody talked of it, everyone was curing incurable diseases with it; but now not a syllable is said upon the subject."[31] Georges Soulié de Morant, a French diplomat resident in China who became fascinated by acupuncture as a cure for cholera and subsequently published his influential book *L'Acupunture Chinoise* in 1939, kindled the first of the twentieth-century waves of interest.

In the United States, acupuncture enjoyed a brief period of popularity during the first half of the nineteenth century, particularly among physicians in the Philadelphia area.[32] In 1826, three local physicians conducted experiments with acupuncture as a possible means of resuscitating drowned people, based on claims by European experimenters that they had successfully revived drowned kittens by inserting acupuncture needles into their hearts. Those same physicians were unable to duplicate those successes and subsequently "gave up in disgust."[33] The 1829 edition of Tavernier's *Elements of Operative Surgery* included three pages on how and when one might perform not only acupuncture but also "electro-acupuncturation."[34] Publications extolling the practice appeared on occasion for the next twenty years.

Although none of the early American accounts of acupuncture make any mention of acupuncture points or meridians, they all claimed substantial success as a result of inserting needles directly into, or in the immediate vicinity of, painful or otherwise afflicted areas. However, by the second half of the nineteenth century, Western practitioners had largely abandoned acupuncture. In 1859 it was concluded that "its advantages have been much overrated, and the practice . . . has fallen into disrepute."[35] The *Index Catalogue* of the Surgeon-General's Library includes barely a half-dozen titles on the subject for the entire half-century of 1850–1900.

THE HISTORY OF VETERINARY ACUPUNCTURE

In contrast to the history of human acupuncture, the history of veterinary acupuncture is somewhat more obscure and has not been extensively studied, but the assertions that acupuncture has been practiced on animals for thousands of years are simply baseless. When compared to the human practice, it is clear that veterinary acupuncture, as currently practiced, is a relatively recent invention.

As in Chinese medicine for humans, the bases of traditional veterinary medicine in China have been described as "imaginary, religious, mystic, and empirical."[36] Within it, there is no evidence that acupuncture, which is unambiguously defined by historians of Chinese medicine as puncturing the skin with needles in association with theories involving *qi* and with the *mai* or "vessels" containing *qi*, was *ever* a historical practice of ancient China. The first Chinese agricultural manual to survive and the first work to contain veterinary material (bits and pieces of information on the treatment of animals) is the sixth-century *Qimin yaoshu*. The text contains nothing remotely resembling acupuncture.[37]

The first recorded veterinary therapeutic tradition involving needling of any sort appears to begin in Song times, perhaps around 1000 A.D. or, more likely, somewhat after. This fact is in contradistinction to what has been published, as well as what appears to have become common knowledge. Indeed, it has been claimed that there is a source called "*Bai-le's Canon of Veterinary Medicine*, [that was] written around 650 B.C., [and] was based primarily on acupuncture," but this statement is totally unsupportable. Although Bo Le, also known as Sun Yang, seems to have been a historical figure who lived in the seventh century B.C. and was said to have been knowledgeable in the "cure of horses," no text known to actually have been written by him is known to exist. Those texts associated with his name first appear in the historical record more than a thousand years after his death. A *Bo Le zhima zabing jing* [*Canon of Bo Le's Treating Various Diseases of Horses*] is one of several veterinary medical texts listed in the bibliographic section of the *Suishu*, the *Official History of the Sui Dynasty* (A.D. 581–618), but the work itself has been lost and the title alone provides few hints as to the methods emphasized. Certainly nothing in the title *Bo Le zhima zabing jing* in any way links the book to acupuncture. In fact, Bo Le himself achieved prominence not as a medical therapist, but as a physiognomist, one skilled in judging the character of the horse from external body features such as hair whorls.[38] In any case, there is no surviving work associated with the name of Bo Le or any kind of needling until the 1384 printing of the *Simu anji ji* [*Collection for Administering the Pasturing and Pacification of Stallions*], which includes a subtext entitled *Bo Le Zhenjing* [*Bo Le's Needling Classic*[39]] devoted almost entirely to bleeding and cauterization (which are, in fact, Eurasian traditions). This was some two thousand years after the death of the historical Bo Le.

Among Song sources calling for the needling of animals is the *Fanmu zuan yanfang* [*Compendium of Efficacious Recipes from the Nomadic Tradition*], compiled by Wang Yu in either the late eleventh or early twelfth century A.D. (although the surviving version is probably based on one from the late thirteenth or early fourteenth century), which deals with camel medicine.[40] Although needling is mentioned, the needling described is very much a minor tradition and is clearly *not* in any way associated with the kind of theoretical underpinnings necessary to call it acupuncture, no matter how one reads this work. Instead, it is mostly cauterization and bleeding, as done in the contemporary West, and as far back as Ancient Greece.

The key works in Chinese veterinary medicine appear later, the most important dating from the seventeenth and eighteenth centuries, and related primarily to horses. The best known is the Ming Dynasty *Yuan Heng liaoma ji* [*Collection for Treating the Horse*]§, published circa 1608 A.D.[41]

In this text, needling is applied in various forms in traditional Chinese veterinary texts, although always strictly secondary to herbal treatments (which are delivered primarily in the form of drenches). However, again, it is clear that this needling, as described in the traditional texts, has essentially nothing to do with modern acupuncture. Instead, needling (*zhen*) appears to refer to *any* intervention with a sharp or hot object. Furthermore, the authors of the *Yuan Heng liaoma ji* clearly distinguish between acupuncture and other human medical traditions and those of veterinary medicine and insist that the relevant points are different between humans and animals.** The points described are used for such interventions as bleeding, surgery, cauterization, or divination—not acupuncture.

In the numerous illustrations in the *Yuan Heng liaoma ji* associated with needling, it is significant that there is no indication of the types of links associating a connected series of points (e.g., conduits or conduit vessels), although there are individual points that are often associated with organs. Otherwise

---

§The *Yuan Heng liaoma ji* has traditionally been attributed to two brothers who may never have existed. The 1608 edition, the first to name them, was not actually the first edition and their names are not associated with earlier editions known from Japanese tradition and implied in the preface to the 1608 edition. Their association with the manual as authors may thus be nothing more than an invention of the publisher, or perhaps Yuan and Heng were simply two individuals putting up money to fund a new edition. There is also the possibility that their names are actually a play on words since Yuan Heng refers to a *Yijing* [*Book of Changes*] passage dealing with horses.

**Guo HuaiXi: *Xinke zhushi ma niu to jing da quan ji* [*Newly Printed and Annotated Horse, Ox, and Camel Classics*], p. 40. Discussion of Po Lo's needling (from the *Simu an ji ji*): Dongxi asked Qu Chuan saying: "I have heard that humans have 360 depressions. Are the needling depressions of horses like this?" Qu Chuan replied saying: "Humans have 360 longitudinal connections [*jing*], horses have 159 'bright temples' [*mingtang*]." Dongxi said: "The five viscera and the like are the same for humans and horses but the needling depressions of horses are not the same as those of humans. Why?" Qu Chuan said: "The human is the divine element among the myriad things. Humans avail of the great movement of *Yin* and *Yang*. They receive the choicest aspects of Heaven and Earth. Their bodies are the proper way of the Five Elements. They receive the primeval influences and become replete and fertile. And they have 360 depressions. They are of the sort that make substantial the revolutions of the absolute according to the 366 days of the calendar year. Now, as for animals, they are things." [All translations are by the authors.]

stated, the points are individual, used for bleeding and/or cauterization, and the theoretical system developed in human acupuncture is entirely lacking. Also apparently lacking is simple needling using very fine "needles" of the type found in human acupuncture (except in a very few surgical interventions, such as cataract removal). Indeed, contemporaneous Japanese sources show needles that look far different from those currently employed in modern acupuncture.[42] Rather than slender, filiform needles, the needles of seventeenth- and eighteenth-century Eastern veterinary literature appear to be lancets or blades, such as would be used for bleeding or lancing abscesses and other lesions. Such needles are even represented in modern literature.[43] The *Yuan Heng liaoma ji* and similar texts thus describe needling (bleeding, lancing, surgery, etc.) traditions that have nothing in common with acupuncture as practiced in human Chinese medicine or in modern veterinary medicine. Instead, the roots of "modern" veterinary acupuncture can be most clearly traced to nineteenth-century Europe.[44]

Much of the historical practice of human and veterinary acupuncture is quite recent and of curious origin. For example, ear acupuncture has been recommended for various procedures in small animal and equine medicine and surgery[45] although it was developed by a French physician P. F. M. Nogier, based on his "sudden intuition" that the antihelix of the ear had to be equated with an upside-down model of the fetal human vertebral column.[46] (Ear acupuncture has also been employed in animals, although the similarity between the shapes of animal ears and their fetuses may be difficult to ascertain.) Acupuncture analgesia, perhaps the most commonly promoted application of the practice, is an invention of the late 1950s.[47] Acupuncture anesthesia, which has been claimed by proponents to be evidence of its effectiveness, is not popular in China and most recently was used for clinical anesthesia in from 0 to 10 percent of cases in ten large Chinese hospitals surveyed in 2001.[48]

Similarly, some of the traditional theoretical aspects of veterinary acupuncture are also modern. For example, the association with and translation of the vital vapor *qi* as a form of energy was not made until 1939, at the same time that the term *meridian* was coined.[49] Animal acupuncture meridians date only to the 1970s and were invented at the insistence of Western practitioners,[50] although even some acupuncture practitioners question their existence. Despite this, various authors (mostly Western) have discovered meridians in cattle, pigs, dogs, cats, and various other species, mostly by "transposition" from one of many human charts.[51] Considered from a historical perspective, such transposition might seem inappropriate in light of the Confucian tradition that the human, civilized world should never mix with that of the savage (animal) one.[52] Indeed, as previously noted, the ancient Chinese made explicit reference that treatment points—whatever the treatment—were not the same in humans as in animals.

Additional modern twists to acupuncture include misinterpreting the common historical and multicultural practice of bleeding at points as "hemo-acupuncture," the injection of aqueous substances at putative points as "aquapuncture," and even the application of colored lights as "colorpuncture." Clinicians in the People's Republic of China introduced local electrical analgesia as part of the acupuncture process in the late 1960s, giving rise to "electroacupuncture."[53] All such techniques appear to have been applied to animals.

Conversely, numerous historical Chinese veterinary practices appear to have been largely abandoned. For example, prohibitions against needling on certain days associated with the 60-day cycle of the traditional Chinese calendar or with phases of the moon appear not to be followed.[54] Similarly, "divination" techniques, whereby through close examination of physical and morphological features such as swirl patterns in the coat, one may determine whether a particular horse will be lucky or unlucky, appear to have lost their historical importance.[55]

Finally, traditional Chinese texts appear to have been regularly misinterpreted in the veterinary literature, leading to a false impression about animal acupuncture history. For example, a chart from the *Yuan Heng liaoma ji* has been claimed to show lateral acupuncture points.[56] However, the accompanying text indicates that such points are, in fact, areas (*jie*—knots) where feces accumulate and cause colic.[57] A subsequent illustration in the original text even shows an arm inserted rectally in an effort to remove the impactions at their source.

An even stranger claim has been advanced with respect to some well-known Chinese *stellae* associated with the foundation of the Tang dynasty in the seventh century. One veterinary author points out that "a sculpture from Tang Dynasty (580–900 C.E.) [sic] Emperor Taizong's tomb is widely purported to be the first illustrated use of acupuncture in horses."[58] Another states that "a rock carving from the Han dynasty [sic] (about 200B.C.) [sic] shows soldiers using arrows to perform acupuncture on their horses to stimulate them before battle."[59]

The rock carvings in question are displayed in the Chinese Rotunda at the University of Pennsylvania's Museum of Archaeology and Anthropology. The reliefs have nothing to do with acupuncture. The following description is available there and on the museum's website.[60]

> The two bas reliefs of horses [from the Tang dynasty] (circa 618–906 A.D.) on the rotunda's west wall were two of six reliefs commissioned by Emperor T'ai-tsung [Taizong]ᶠ, founder of the T'ang [Tang] Dynasty, for his mausoleum. The portraits of the six favorite horses T'ai-tsung had ridden in his battles to secure the empire's borders are

well known in Chinese history and literature. Each horse is identified by the position of its arrow wound. The pictured relief shows General Ch'iu Hsing-kung [Qiu Xinggong], who had given up his own unwounded horse to the Emperor, pulling an arrow from the chest of Autumn Dew, the Emperor's wounded charger.

A philological approach to Chinese veterinary medicine, with accurate translations from original source material, is sorely needed in approaching the history of acupuncture. A historian of medicine, D. C. Epler, Jr., has observed: "The technique [acupuncture] is said to be over 2,000 years old and contemporary authors continue to cite ancient texts when describing its theoretical foundations. However, when these ancient texts are approached as historical documents, rather than as source books that can be continually reinterpreted for medical practitioners, then they indicate vast differences between the early use of needles and the present form of acupuncture. What is now known as acupuncture is thus the result of a long development and bears little resemblance to its ancestral version." So it is with the putative history of veterinary acupuncture. In fact, claims for the extreme antiquity of human and veterinary acupuncture are widely reported in the veterinary acupuncture literature but are not supported by the historical record.[61]

CHIROPRACTIC

Manipulation of the spine and other joints is a medical practice that can be traced to early medical practitioners of various civilizations, including Greek, Chinese, and American Indian. During the seventeenth and eighteenth centuries, English "bonesetters" based their practices on the belief that little bones could move out of place (and could be put back in place with an audible "click").[62] Osteopathy was founded in 1874 and was initially based partly on the theory that misplaced spinal bones obstructed the flow and balance of bodily fluids. Various manipulative techniques are currently employed by a variety of practitioners of human care, including osteopathic physicians, physical therapists, medical doctors, and chiropractors.

Of the therapies promoted as alternative, the history of chiropractic (from Greek *cheir* [hands] and *praxis* [act or motion]) manipulation, which is sometimes referred to as "adjusting," is the most recent and the most well documented. The original theories and practices of chiropractic can be directly traced back to the Canadian-born Daniel David Palmer.

Palmer initially acknowledged the historical foundations of his several theories of chiropractic (Palmer's theories underwent considerable change over the 17 years that he practiced chiropractic) but went on to credit the experience he gained during nine years of practice as a magnetic healer in the 1880s and '90s for their ultimate formation.[63] Noting the long and unsuccessful history of available therapeutic methods, including "herbs, barks and roots for medicinal use" and "powders, ointments, pills, elixirs, decoctions, tinctures and lotions of all known vegetables and crawling creatures," Palmer became interested in searching for the cause of disease. Palmer reported that he cured two people—one who was deaf and the other suffering from "heart trouble"— by replacing a displaced vertebra that was purported to be pressing against nerves. Noting the disparate nature of the conditions but asserting a similar underlying pathology, for Palmer, the amount of "nerve tension" became the single cause of all disease. What particular kind of disease afflicted a patient depended on what nerves were "too tense or too slack" and whether there was "an excess or deficiency of functionating [sic]."[64]

Palmer's theories were also vitalistic. As with many other historical approaches to healing, he subscribed to the notion of a vital force or spirit. He stated, "Spirit soul and body compose the being, the source of mentality. Innate and Educated, two mentalities, look after the welfare of the body physically and its surrounding environments." Thus, he concluded that "the dualistic system—spirit and body—united by intellectual life—the soul—is the basis of this science of biology, and nerve tension is the basis of functional activity in health and disease." In order to correct the problems that Palmer identified, he "created the art of adjusting vertebrae, using the spinous and transverse processes as levers, and named the mental act of accumulating knowledge, the cumulative function, corresponding to the physical vegetative function—growth of intellectual and physical—together, with the science, art and philosophy—Chiropractic."

Over time, Palmer's theories underwent considerable change, perhaps in response to the criticism that his initial theories received from the medical and osteopathic professions, as well as from his own graduates. By 1903, he had given up his initial theories, which held that displacement of *any* anatomic part could lead to inflammation and disease, replacing those with the idea that bones out of place caused disease, resulting in a pinching of nerves.

The concept that bones out of place could cause disease resulted in the term that still defines the chiropractic profession, the "subluxation." Adopted in 1903 by S. M. Langworthy, a former student and subsequent rival of Palmer's, the subluxation has formed the basis for chiropractic authority while at the same time it has been the source of its greatest controversy. This controversy exists because, on the one hand, chiropractors have been legally defined as those who diagnose and treat subluxations, but on the other hand, such an anatomical lesion has never been demonstrated, at least in any sense used by the chiropractic profession. Indeed, it has been recently stated that "evaluation of the chiropractic lesion(s) remains perhaps the greatest frustration and challenge facing researchers and S/Ps [scientist/practitioners] alike. Quantitative and qualitative definition of the phases of VSC [vertebral subluxation complex], SDF [segmental dysfunction], and RDF [regional dysfunction] are needed, and no operational definition of even a most Generic 'manipulable lesion' is available at this time."[65]

The reliance on a nondemonstrable lesion as the cause of all disease set up the chiropractic profession as a target for the scientific biomedical community. Nevertheless, over time, by political, legal, and social machinations, the chiropractic profession has been able to secure its legal status to practice on humans, and has even won a major restraint of trade lawsuit[††] against the American Medical Association.[66] Still, neither the chiropractic subluxation, nor any other defined entity, nor a physiologic mechanism of action by which spinal adjustments might work, has ever been accurately, or even consistently, defined.

The current state of chiropractic practice and philosophy shows vast differences among practitioners. Some in the field still ascribe to traditional Palmerian theories while others have advocated a scientific approach to evaluation of the therapies and have abandoned the subluxation.[67] However, as chiropractors abandon subluxations and adopt procedures commonly used in other disciplines, such as physical therapy, or even acupuncture and homeopathy, they face increasing market competition and have responded to such competition by attempting to gain legislative authority over use of manipulative techniques.

Veterinary Chiropractic

Apparently no formal attempts were made in the early years of chiropractic to introduce its theories into veterinary medicine, although a blank diploma for an "Equine Adjustor" can be found in the Palmer Archives in Iowa. However, early chiropractors may have tried to use chiropractic on animals. For example, in 1921, two horses with azoturia[‡‡] ("in effect it acts like a paralysis") were reportedly cured with chiropractic manuevers.[68] In 1923, a chiropractic school publication published a letter called, "Pigs have backbones with Subluxations that Adjustments work On" and described the treatment of two partially paralyzed pigs.[69] D. D. Palmer's son, B. J. Palmer, perhaps the most important

---

[††]In 1987, federal court judge Susan Getzendanner concluded that during the 1960s "there was a lot of material available to the AMA Committee on Quackery that supported its belief that all chiropractic was unscientific and deleterious." The judge also noted that chiropractors still took too many X rays. However, she ruled that the AMA had engaged in an illegal boycott. She concluded that the dominant reason for the AMA's antichiropractic campaign was the belief that chiropractic was not in the best interest of patients. But she ruled that this did not justify attempting to contain and eliminate an entire licensed profession without first demonstrating that a less-restrictive campaign could not succeed in protecting the public. Although chiropractors trumpet the antitrust ruling as an endorsement of their effectiveness, the case was decided on narrow legal grounds (restraint of trade) and was not an evaluation of chiropractic methods. (Reprinted, with permission, http//www.chirobase.org.)

[‡‡]Modern terminology would describe azoturia as exertional rhabdomyolysis.

figure in advancing chiropractic in its early days, apparently maintained a "veterinarian" [sic] hospital where vertebral subluxations of cows, horses, cats, dogs, and other animals were adjusted. Palmer asserted that the application of chiropractic principles was the same, whether applied to humans or animals. Paradoxically, many chiropractors felt that downplaying animal applications of chiropractic was prudent, lest the public begin to call them "horse doctors,"[70] the term being one of opprobrium at the time. In 1957, an article noted that adjustments had been made on cattle, dogs, and a pig "suffering from such diverse conditions as foot rot, shipping fever, lumpy jaw, acute indigestion, etc., with improvement or complete recovery in all but two patients."[60] Chiropractic approaches to veterinary problems were featured in a chiropractic journal in the 1980s,[71] with one two-part article even stating that "veterinary" chiropractic "proved the chiropractic premise"![72]

Skeptical responses to applications of chiropractic philosophy to veterinary medicine appear sporadically throughout history, as well. For example, an advertisement of a chiropractic school appealing to "veterinarians who are desirous of retiring from veterinary practice," appeared in a 1923 veterinary journal, prompting this acerbic comment: "It is to be doubted whether a successful veterinarian who had the means and mood to retire would care to top off his career by bursting forth as a chiropractor. . . . The intention may be to address primarily the veterinarian who simply wants to quit and seek another way of making a living. . . . If he had been an able and conscientious practitioner of veterinary medicine, he would be too strongly imbued with the more thorough principles of his science ever to feel at ease as an apostle of drugless healing . . . his head would falter on the spinal column of his patient and he would long to administer the forbidden pill."[73] In 1923 in an article critical of chiropractic, the American Journal of Clinical Medicine used a cartoon to caricature the idea that chiropractic could be applied to horses.[74]

More formal attempts to organize chiropractic practice in animals have been most recently conducted primarily under the auspices of the American Veterinary Chiropractic Association since the late 1970s. The organization certifies both doctors of chiropractic and veterinarians to adjust animals. Current publications by veterinarians attribute both pathology and treatment efforts at subluxations[75,76] or, alternatively, to the vertebral subluxation complex,[77] although such terminology is as vague and ill defined in the veterinary field as it is in the human field. The AVCA has also lobbied for recognition as a profession separate from veterinary medicine or human chiropractic.

HOMEOPATHY

The German physician Samuel Hahnemann (1755–1843) is generally acknowledged to be the founder and developer of homeopathy, although some of his concepts appear very early in medical history. Hahnemann had a formal medical education but appears never to have practiced medicine regularly.

Early in his career, Hahnemann apparently became dissatisfied with the state of medicine. At the time, "heroic" medicine included bleeding ("the living human body may, perhaps, never have contained one drop of blood too much"), purging, cupping, blisters, cathartics ("so many attempts to remove a hostile material principle which never did and never could have existed"), and excessive doses of mercury. He became a strong critic of contemporary medical practices, particularly their "imaginary and supposed material cause of disease."[78] He was also a vocal critic of contemporary pharmacological and pharmaceutical practices, and noted that the drugs available at that time were prescribed without an experimental knowledge of their effects, and were often compounded incorrectly and haphazardly.[79]

Hahnemann followed the tradition that viewed disease as a matter of the "vital force" or spirit. The concept of the vital force or spirit, the alleged nonmaterial force that sustains life and for which there is no objective evidence,[80] is one of the earliest speculations in recorded medical history and similar forces form the proposed basis for any number of metaphysical health practices (e.g., *qi* in acupuncture or the "innate" of chiropractic). According to Hahnemann, "The causes of our maladies cannot be material, since the least foreign material substance, however mild it may appear to us, if introduced into our blood-vessels, is promptly ejected by the vital force, as though it were a poison. . . . [N]o disease, in a word, is caused by any material substance, but that every one is only and always a peculiar, virtual, dynamic derangement of the health."[81]

Consistent with this philosophy was the belief that it is more important to pay attention to symptoms than to any external causes of disease. Knowing the specific symptoms of illness, treatment then became a matter of finding a substance or substances that induced the same symptoms in a healthy individual. This was the basis of the Principle of Similars, which was embraced by Hahnemann. However, as speculation about natural ways of healing goes, like cures like was not exactly new. Hippocrates advocated the concept, so did the Romans (who, for example, advocated raw dog's liver to ward off rabies), and later, and more vocally, so did the Swiss physician and mystic Paracelsus.

Hahnemann initially tested nondiluted remedies such as sulfuric acid and strychnine on his patients, with predictably disastrous results. Somewhat suddenly, Hahnemann modified his principles, most likely because, as a meticulous observer, he was aware of the problems caused by his undiluted remedies. This was most likely the impetus for him to begin decreasing the dosages employed, by diluting the original substance.[82] Ironically, the later work of Pasteur and Koch on inoculations with very small amounts of weakened disease-causing microbes seemed to add support to the notion that diluted substances could cause beneficial effects.

Hahnemann found—predictably, in hindsight—that by diluting his original, sometimes noxious, substances, he could reduce the occurrence of side effects. Hahnemann used a process of sequential dilutions, for example, adding one part of the original substance to one hundred parts of water (C dilution) or 1:10 (D dilution), and then repeating the process over and over, using one part of the new dilution with another ten or one hundred parts of diluent. It is easy to achieve extreme dilutions by this method, dilutions that exceed the point where no molecule of the original substance is likely to remain in the solution (the dilution limit). Hahnemann was most likely unaware that his preparations exceeded the dilution limit.

However, for Hahnemann and homeopathy, simple dilution of a drug was insufficient to produce a cure. It would also be necessary to make the dilutions more powerful through a process known as "potentization." The origin of the principle of potentization is more obscure. According to Hahnemann: "Homeopathic potentizations are processes by which the medicinal properties of drugs, which are in a latent state in the crude substance, are excited and enabled to act spiritually upon the vital forces."[83] Potentization purports to make the diluted, inert substance active by releasing its "energy." To achieve potentization, after each successive 1-to-10 (D) or 1-to-100 (C) dilution, the solution needed to be shaken vigorously (the process is known as "succussion") and then rapped against a hard surface; Hahnemann himself insisted that the surface be a leather-bound book. In the case of a powdered substance, the substance needed to be vigorously ground up (trituration). The energy thus "liberated" by these processes purportedly remains, even in doses at which no single molecule of the originally diluted substance remains (>12 C or >24 D). Such energy is reportedly also able to be transmitted from solutions to the lactose tablet formulations of some homeopathic medications,[84] and, more recently, to be digitized and even transmitted over the internet.[85]

Hahnemann and his followers went on to test the effects of almost one hundred substances on themselves, a process known as "proving" (from the German *Prüfung*). Materials tested were seemingly endless, and included table salt (*natrum muriatum*—most homeopathic remedies are given Latin names), snake venom (*lachesis*), head lice (*Pediculus capitis*), and poison ivy (*Rhus toxicodendron*). The typical procedure was for a healthy person to ingest a small amount of a particular substance and then attempt to note, with meticulous detail, any reaction or symptom (including emotional or mental reactions) that occurred, and attribute those symptoms, no matter how trivial, to ingestion of the remedy. By this method, Hahnemann and his followers proved that the substance was an effective remedy for a particular symptom. Such a method of determining the effects of the medications was condemned almost from its inception, as was the veracity of the results themselves.[86]

Nevertheless, the collected experiences of such incidents became the basis for a compendium called the *Materia Medica*.

These experiences were, to contemporary critics, a compilation of inanities. Lists of symptoms ran from 10 to 50 pages long for each drug, and included such effects as "easily falls asleep when reading," "excessive liability to become pregnant," and "excessive trembling of the body, when dallying with females."[87] Nevertheless, these minute details were exactly the sort of thing that homeopaths viewed as the distinguishing virtue of their approach.

Hahnemann believed that homeopathic remedies must be appropriately prescribed for individual body types and personalities, based on the ancient humoral theories of Galen. According to these theories, there were four body types and personalities, based on which body "humor" predominated: blood (sanguine, warm-hearted, and volatile), black bile (melancholic, sad), yellow bile (choleric, quick to anger and to action), and phlegm (phlegmatic, sluggish, and apathetic). He later suggested that there are a corresponding few primary causes of acute and chronic illnesses, which he called "miasms." The first miasm, known as "psora," (itch) refers to a general susceptibility to disease and may be considered the source of all chronic diseases. The other two miasms in homeopathic theory are the venereal diseases syphilis and sycosis (gonorrhea). Together, these three conditions were considered to be the cause of at least 80 percent of all chronic diseases.[88]

Criticism of the practice of homeopathy came from inside and outside of the field. The regular medical profession, led by the poet-physician Oliver Wendell Holmes, reacted to homeopathy with scorn and ridicule, noting, for example, the absurdity of the concept of extreme dilutions by pointing out that by the seventeenth dilution, the homeopath would have added alcohol to the original substance in an amount equivalent to ten thousand Adriatic Seas. Still, "Trifling errors must be expected, but they are as likely to be on one side as the other, and any little matter like Lake Superior or the Caspian would be but a drop in the bucket."[89] The Rhode Island Medical Society offered a fifty dollar prize for the best critique of homeopathy, and the winner wrote, "When things are exceedingly laughable, it is a little unreasonable to demand of us an imperturbable gravity."[90] Even prominent homeopaths, while accepting the law of similars, found Hahnemann's conceptions of the mechanisms of action of homeopathic medications to be "vague, incomplete and even erroneous."[91] Controversy also raged between high- and low-dilution proponents, the latter of whom often disregarded Hahnemann's laws.[92] Hahnemann himself decried dilutions in excess of 30C, saying, "There must be some end to the thing. It cannot go on to infinity."[93]

Later in the nineteenth century, as contemporary orthodox medicine abandoned its extreme practices in favor of more effective and safer therapeutics, and as practicing homeopaths began to accept conventional medical practices, the field weakened. In the early twentieth century, homeopathic colleges, whose graduates were unable to meet the educational standards of medical schools, collapsed. In the 1930s, the Third Reich of Nazi Germany attempted to validate homeopathy under the banner of *Neue Deutsche Heilkunde* [New German Healthcare], however, the results of its research, now lost, seem to have been negative.[94] In addition, while the new scientific medicine experienced revolutionary changes resulting in dramatic improvements in disease management, homeopathy remained relatively stagnant. By the 1960s, the practice of homeopathy had virtually been abandoned,[95] only to reappear with the latest emergence of alternative medicine.

Homeopathy did make several important indirect contributions to the practice of medicine. At the time that it was developed, the medical treatments of the time, such as therapeutic phlebotomy and administration of calomel (mercury salts) were often more dangerous than the disease that they purported to treat. Homeopathy may have helped hasten the demise of such treatments and helped increase recognition that many acute conditions will spontaneously resolve. Homeopathy provided the initial idea and source for useful drugs such as nitroglycerin[96] and aconite.[97] Early scientists such as Joseph Lister and Sidney Ringer stated that they were led to important pharmacological discoveries because of homeopathy.[98] Homeopathy has also been given credit for providing early support for clinical trials with control groups, systematic and quantitative procedures and the use of statistics in medicine.[99] Finally, the apparent successes attributed to the medications may also reinforce and remind medical practitioners of the amazing capacity of the body to heal itself.

Veterinary Homeopathy

Hahnemann did none of his original work on animals, although he apparently had great respect for "veterinary surgeons."[100] The short-lived historical heyday of veterinary homeopathy came in the mid–nineteenth century. The first known homeopathic veterinarian, J. J. W. Lux, edited a veterinary homeopathy journal in the 1830s.[101] Scottish graduate William Haycock published his *Elements of Veterinary Homeopathy* in 1852. To his credit, Haycock was one of the first veterinarians to abandon the practice of therapeutic bleeding.[102] J. C. Schaeffer published his *New Manual of Homoeopathic Veterinary Medicine* in 1863, stating, "The blessings of Homoeopathy [*sic*] are no longer the exclusive property of man; the irrational brute has become the partaker of this great gift of God to his creatures."[103] Interestingly, Schaeffer's work was intended to "enable every owner of domestic animals to treat them himself without being obliged to send to a distant city for a veterinary surgeon."[104] Such intent would not seem unreasonable even today, given that homeopathic remedies are prescribed to treat easily recognized symptoms and not disease.

How homeopathy could be directly applied to animals was never explained. It would seem particularly difficult to determine symptomatology such as "frightful dreams about falling from a height" by examining an animal; in general, the fallacy of prescribing medications for animals based on how those medications make people feel seems somewhat difficult to rationalize, given obvious interspecies variations between reactions to various pharmacological substances. The concepts of prescribing medications for body types and personalities would seem to be particularly difficult to apply to animals, as well, although concerns about transmission of psora to animals from humans have been recently expressed.[105]

At the turn of the twentieth century, interest in veterinary applications of homeopathic principles was on the decline. Historical criticisms of veterinary homeopathy were similar to those espoused in human medicine and are as salient today. For example: "No curative system directing its efforts, as homeopathy does, merely against the symptoms of disease can ever rest on a safe or scientific basis . . . Not only are the principles upon which homeopathy are said to based untenable, but the details of the system are inconsistent and ridiculous."[106] Despite such criticisms, and the decline of homeopathy throughout most of the twentieth century,[107] the practice has enjoyed some resurgence. In the United States, recent efforts at a revival of the practice have been sparked by such organizations as the American Holistic Veterinary Association and the Association of Homeopathic Veterinarians.

HERBAL AND BOTANICAL THERAPIES

As far back as evidence can be gathered, humans used various medicinal plants (along with magic and religious tenets) to treat their ailments, and presumably, those of their animals. Some evidence for their use dates back to the Neanderthal period.[108] Prescriptions for the use of various plants can be found in the medical lexicon of virtually every society in recorded history. In the sixteenth century, medical schools created botanical gardens to grow medicinal plants.[109] The importation of medicinal plants from central and South America had a profound impact on the therapeutics of sixteenth- and seventeenth-century Europe.[110] Until the twentieth century, most remedies were botanicals, a few of which were found—through trial and error—to be helpful. American housewives of the colonial period would gather plants and wild herbs and hang them to dry for future use, although the types of herbs generally used, such as sarsaparilla, horehound, and dandelion, in reality could neither hurt nor help.[111]

More formal programs involving the use of herbal and botanical remedies also arose. For example, in the United States, between 1836 and 1911, 13 physio-medical colleges, which substituted botanical medicines for pharmaceutical drugs and which promoted the belief in the ubiquitous vital force, opened and then closed their doors.[112] Similarly, the Thomsonian movement of the mid-1800s found great popularity by emphasizing herbal remedies (in addition to steaming the body to overcome the "power" of cold). However, the influence of these, and other, medical sects, waned as they could no longer match the advances of science and the resulting public trust that accompanied those advances.

The active ingredients of some pharmaceuticals in widespread use today are identical to, or derivatives of, bioactive constituents of historic folk remedies. Herbal and botanical sources form the origin of as much as 30 percent of all modern pharmaceuticals.[113] Aspirin (acetylsalicylic acid) is a derivative of salicylic acid, which, as salicin (salicyl alcohol plus a sugar molecule), occurs in the flower buds of the meadowsweet (spirea) and in the bark and leaves of several poplars and willows, notably the white willow (*Salix alba*). White-willow-bark extracts were used for centuries as a pain remedy. Indeed, Hippocrates reportedly prescribed willow bark and leaves for fever and the pain of childbirth. And in many cultures, soaked willow leaves have been used as a topical painkiller. Digoxin is a derivative of foxglove, of which there are at least 12 varieties. Historically, purple foxglove was found to be helpful for "dropsy" (congestive heart failure). Quinine was an important antipyretic, first isolated from cinchona bark in 1820. As it became inexpensive and widely available, it was employed for the treatment of fever of virtually any origin. The use of quinine became so widespread in the days after the Civil War that the AMA tried unsuccessfully to convince the federal government to grow the tree in the United States.[114]

However, the historical use of botanicals—even the existence of pharmacologically active ingredients in some of them—may also obscure real problems. Salicin, the parent of salicylate drugs, was first isolated in the last century. But to ingest 1 gram of salicin, only about half as potent as aspirin, from willow bark, one would have to ingest at least 14 grams of the bark. The tannins in willow bark, as well as salicin are very irritating to the stomach; however, while unacceptable today, severe side effects were an acknowledged part of historical medical therapy.[115] According to detailed descriptions from historical texts, all 12 varieties of digitalis plants had active compounds of varying qualities, with the seeds having at least six different biologically active chemical variations, showing cardiac, as well as other effects. Potency deteriorated after a number of months even when the preparations were kept hermetically sealed. The different compounds had various absorption rates from the gastrointestinal tract and there were variations from batch to batch depending on growing conditions.[116]

In the 1880s, research with coal tars led to the development of synthetic antipyretics, which quickly took quinine's place. The trend from crude to synthesized pharmaceuticals has continued, but due to the obvious fact that some herbal and botanical remedies contain pharmacologically active ingredients, the development of drugs from plants continues, and many drug companies are engaged in large-scale pharmacological screening of herbs.

Historical usage notwithstanding, popular herbalism (with its slogan of "botanicals are safer") appears to have abandoned most of the obvious pharmacologically active herbs (such as belladonna, ergot, and colchicum) to the pharmaceutical industry, since their therapeutic window is so narrow and misuse can be deadly.[117] Those that remain in more common use are likely to have neither the therapeutic potency nor the toxicity profile of botanicals such as foxglove.

In addition, the current usage of botanicals is quite different from their historical use. Historically, herbs may have served to placate the patient, and perhaps even helped to relieve some symptoms. However, at the same time herbs were used in smaller amounts, as specific treatments (rather than prophylactically, in order to prevent health problems), in crude form (as opposed to enriched extracts), and not in association with other synthetic medications (obviating concerns about herb-drug interactions).[118]

The historical successes attributed to botanicals also carried a cost. The indications for using a given botanical were poorly defined. Dosages were, unavoidably, arbitrary because the concentrations of the active ingredient were unknown. Any number of contaminants may have been present. Most important, many of the remedies simply did not work, and some were harmful or even deadly. There was no effective way of conveying useful information; herbalists copied extensively from one another over millennia and mixed accurate (by modern standards) information with nonsense, misconceptions, and inaccuracies. The only way to separate the beneficial from the useless or hazardous was through anecdotes relayed mainly by word of mouth.[119] The true identities of the plants used are doubtful, in regard to both genus and species. Furthermore, the societal acceptability of risk in the treatment of disease was higher.[120] Accordingly, it may not be possible to use the historical record as a guide for many of the currently advocated uses of herbal and botanical products.

Veterinary Herbal and Botanical Medicine

The history of veterinary applications of herbals and botanicals is nearly as long and well documented as it is in human medicine.[121] For example, black and white hellebore (*Helleborus niger* and *Veratrum album*, respectively) were inserted through the ear of horses or sheep by Pliny in the first century A.D., and were used in the early twentieth century as a purgative, emetic, anthelmintic, and parasiticide (although it caused death in many animals). Historical prescriptions for herbal use can be found in such diverse sources as the Chinese *Yuan Heng liaoma ji* and in the medicinal practices of the North American Indian.[122] Botanical horse medicines were provided during the Civil War.[123] Even as late as 1957, popular books continued to list such substances as aconite, belladonna, cinchone, ipecac, nux vomica (strychnine), and tobacco for veterinary use.[124] However, more recently, such titles were in scant evidence until the latest revival of interest in the use of herbal and botanical veterinary remedies.[125]

ELECTRICAL AND MAGNETIC THERAPY

Electricity and magnetism have apparently had a place in the popular imagination and medical treatment for more than three thousand years, although their importance has waxed and waned over time. The time and place of the discovery of electricity and magnetism, much less their first therapeutic use, is unknown. However, the effects of these agents have most likely been studied and debated since their use was first described.

Pliny the Elder (23–79A.D.) wrote in his *Natural History* that about a thousand years previously, a shepherd, in what is now Turkey, noted that the iron nails in his sandals were pulled to the ground. This attraction supposedly led him to discover stones that contained the attractive forces. The rocks were originally named magnesian (from Magnes, the shepherd's name) or lode (course, point) stones. The invisible power of magnets led to fanciful stories: magnetic islands that could hold ships with iron nails stationary (Ptolemy, 100–200A.D. in his *Geography*) and even destroy them by pulling their nails out (*The Arabian Knights*—The Tale of the Third Beggar).[126]

At the same time, it was also known that substances such as amber, when rubbed with fur, could attract small objects; electric rays (capable of generating >200 volts) were used for maladies such as gout and headache.[127] Various parts of electric fish were long advocated as folk medicine, to be taken orally or applied locally, and were studied by numerous investigators including Galen; such investigations continued until well into the nineteenth century.[128] Some cultures were still using electric fish at least into the mid–twentieth century.[129]

Magnets were the subject of numerous theories about life and healing. For example, Thales of Miletus (636?–546?B.C.) taught that the essence of life was related to the ability to move. Because magnets and electrostatic substances such as amber can cause iron and small bits of cloth and paper to move, Thales concluded that they also have lifelike characteristics—a magical association not unlike that proposed in early Chinese medicine. By 200 A.D., Greek

"Electrical and Magnetic Therapy" was written with Jeffrey Basford, MD, PhD. Some material reprinted from J. R. Basford, A historical perspective of the popular use of electric and magnetic therapy (*Arch Phys Med Rehabil* 2001; 82[9]: 1261–69; with permission from Elsevier Science).

healers used amber pills to stop bleeding and magnetic rings as a treatment for arthritis.

In 1289, Peter Peregrinus[130] noted that when a small needle was placed in various positions on the surface of a spherical piece of lodestone, contour lines of force could be described that converged at two opposing locations. Peregrinus named these points of convergence the north and south "poles." He also postulated that magnetic forces might be harnessed to produce mechanical energy (i.e., an electric motor) and may have been the first European to explain how a magnetic needle might be used as a compass. (Perhaps even more remarkable is the fact that Peregrinus did not attribute magnetism to mystical or godlike forces, rather, he used a scientific method.)

By the end of the Middle Ages, magnets were used to retrieve foreign bodies such as iron knife blades and arrowheads from the body.[131] In addition, it was widely believed that magnets had wondrous powers and were useful as aphrodisiacs and for curing baldness, for wound "purification," and for the treatment of arthritis and gout. Chaucer, Bacon, and Shakespeare all allude to the attractive powers of magnets.[132,133]

Paracelsus (1493–1542) investigated the effects of magnets on epilepsy, diarrhea, and hemorrhage and believed that humans attracted good and evil in the same way that iron responds to a magnetic field. He also believed that the two magnetic poles had different effects, for example, he recommended that the south pole of a magnet be held near the head and the north pole near the abdomen of people with epilepsy to "push" and "pull" the disease from the body. Spurious claims for differing clinical effects of magnetic poles may even by made today.

In the sixteenth century, differences between magnetic forces and electrostatic attractions were first described. Studies by Cardano (1501–1576), an Italian mathematician and physician, led to the belief that all matter contains "humours" and that changes in their concentration cause substances to be attracted or repelled (the Roman poet Lucretius had made similar claims 1,500 years earlier). William Gilbert (1544–1603) introduced the term *electricity*, derived from *ilektron*, the Greek word for amber.[134] Gilbert's work spread to France and Italy and influenced famous early scientists such as Bruno, Galileo, and Descartes.

Scientific interest in electricity and magnetism was mirrored by the general public's interest in magnetism and magnetic cures. An English physician, Thomas Browne (1605–1682), wrote *Pseudodoxia Epidemica* [*Inquiries into Vulgar and Common Errors*] in which he attempted to dispassionately examine medical and popular beliefs and traditions, including magnetism. Browne disproved long-standing beliefs that diamonds can weaken, and that garlic can destroy, magnetic fields. Browne also pointed out that any effects that magnetic salves might have might be due to the chemical properties of the medium, and the magnetic material that was mixed in it, rather than from magnetism itself. He attributed the use of magnetic amulets to treat diseases such as gout, headaches, and venereal disease to wishful thinking.

Otto von Guericke constructed the first electrostatic apparatus in 1650, although he did not recognize static electricity as such.[135] The first electrostatic generator was invented in the early 1700s by a protégé of Newton's, Francis Hauksbee,[136] and led to an increased practicality of electrical study and demonstration. Hauksbee and others began "electric boy" demonstrations in which a small boy was insulated from the ground and charged with a static electricity generator. In these displays, electricity was passed on to other people; that sparks could be drawn from the boy if a conductor was brought toward him and that he attracted small bits of paper or feathers in the same way that a piece of charged amber did.[137]

By the mid-1700s, similar electrostatic developments were taking place in Germany. In 1744, Kratzenstein was one of the first to apply "artificial" electricity to medicine. A year or two later, in Leyden, a device was created that would both generate and store large quantities of electric charge. This became known as the Leyden jar and was used in experiments with plants and animals.[138]

In the New World, Benjamin Franklin, intrigued by an exposition in Boston, began studying electricity, discovering the basic principles of electrostatics and developing terminology (*charge, discharge, condenser, battery, electrical shock, electrician, positive, negative, plus,* and *minus*) still used today. He also studied the therapeutic effects of electricity, for example, experimenting with electric shocks as a cure for paralysis. He noted that while paralyzed limbs appeared to gain strength and move on a temporary basis, effects were transient and the patients went home discouraged. Others noted the numbing paresthesias produced by electrical machines.[139] Many were swept along in the new tide of electrotherapy, and it was accepted as useful for the treatment of paralysis, poor circulation of body fluids, irregular operation of "the principle of life," and even decreased perspiration.[140]

Concurrent with Franklin's investigations, an Austrian physician, Franz Anton Mesmer (1734–1815), was producing medical cures with magnetized pieces of iron. (With time he found that substances such as paper, wool, silk, and even human beings, which had no magnetic properties, were also effective.)[141] Mesmer believed the cures stemmed from a combination of gravitational and magnetic forces that he named "animal magnetism."[142] Mesmer believed that if a sick person were exposed to a magnetic field (i.e., mesmerized—Mesmer also became enthralled with hypnotism, and today the term *mesmerized* is often used as a synonym for hypnotized), he or she would undergo a "crisis" and emerge cured (parallels with the "healing crisis" described by homeopaths are perhaps obvious). Mesmerism and Mesmer became wildly popular with everyone but Austria's medical establishment.

Failing to cure a child pianist and favorite of Queen Maria Theresa, Mesmer moved to Paris where he became a center of controversy as he had been in Vienna. Finally, Louis XVI established a commission to investigate Mesmerism that included Guillotine (the inventor of the guillotine), Lavoisier, and Benjamin Franklin. No evidence of biophysical (in distinction to "curative") activity was found, and Mesmer's treatments were ruled to be fraudulent.[143,144,]

Despite Mesmer's failure, interest in the electricity, magnetism, and non-traditional cures continued in the United States. Thus, by 1795, Elisha Perkins, a Connecticut physician and apparent mule trader, developed devices that he claimed "draw off the noxious electrical fluid that lay at the root of suffering."[145] These "magnetic attractors" (also known as "tractors") consisted of pairs of small wedges made from metallic alloys (e.g., copper, zinc, and gold or iron, silver, and platinum). Perkins obtained a patent for his tractors and became a rich man despite charges from the Connecticut Medical Society that he was a fraud. Perkins, however, apparently believed in his treatments as he died of yellow fever while providing tractor treatment during a 1799 New York epidemic. Elisha's son, Benjamin, took the magnetic tractors to England, where they were met with similar initial success. The magnetic tractors were eventually discredited, but Benjamin Perkins left England a very wealthy man.

Hans Christian Oerstad discovered the relation of electricity and magnetism in 1820 when he observed that a flowing current deflected a compass needle and that a magnet could exert a force on a wire carrying electric current. Within the next 45 years, Michael Faraday discovered that a magnetic field could induce a current in a moving wire and James Clerk Maxwell had derived the electromagnetic field equations used today. The development of the electric battery ("pile") and the resultant development of the induction apparatus provided further momentum for electromedical applications.[146]

A physician from Philadelphia was the first to describe the relief of dental pain by electricity, producing analgesia during a tooth extraction by applying one electrode to the "offending tooth" while the patient held the other in his or her hand.[147] The Pennsylvania Association of Dental Surgeons appointed a committee to study the use of electricity in dentistry, reported equivocal results, and therefore did not recommend it for general use.[148] Nonetheless, the technique spread rapidly through both the United States and Europe.

In 1858, W. G. Oliver, an American physician, experimented with electrodes placed on the limbs to produce surgically useful anesthesia and used it to remove an ulcer from the left leg of a male patient.[149] Concurrent demonstrations of electroanesthesia were given in England.[150] However, the new technique was controversial, and a special conference of the College of Dentists in London in 1858 declared that electricity was not an anesthetic agent, that it can augment pain, that it sometimes modifies sensation, and that when favorable results were produced, it was due to "diversion" and not to true

insensibility. Subsequent commissions, in England, as well as France, concluded that electricity was not an effective anesthetic. Electroanesthesia soon lost
popularity and lapsed into obscurity, to be discovered, forgotten, and rediscovered many times subsequently.

Electro-medicine was particularly prominent in the Midwest following the
American Civil War. Alternative treatments flourished in this region. Traveling
salesmen and healers sold a variety of magnetic salves and liniments.[151] Adver-
tisements of the period were speckled with electromagnetic health aids such as
electric rings and magnetic insoles.

Among the colorful figures of late nineteenth century magnetic medicine
was C. J. Thatcher who, for example, wore a magnetic cap, waistcoat, stocking
liners, and insoles while being interviewed by a journalist. He stated: "I can
cure anything. . . . Let the authorities turn over 10 cases to me. I'll put my magnetic shields on 'em and restore the harmonious vibrations of the brain and
everything will be well! Paralysis? An easy problem. Had 5 cases . . . cured 'em
right off." Thatcher's magnetic healing doctrines were based on the belief that
blood's iron content made it the body's most important magnetic conductor
and that disease occurred when the body's ability to gain magnetic power from
the atmosphere was compromised. As has been the current and historical
practice of virtually every promoter of unusual medical claims, Thatcher
attacked the skeptical medical establishment by saying that it resisted his findings out of selfishness.

By the 1890s, a number of scientific papers and books supported a role
for electromagnetic therapy in medicine. For example, investigators at La
Salpêtrière, the French hospital made famous by the pioneer in neurology, Dr.
Jean Martin Charcot (1825–1893), reported that infectious diseases such as
cholera were susceptible to magnetic treatment, and that magnetic fields
could increase "the resistance to conduction in the motor nerves" and were
beneficial in the treatment of hemiparesis. These reports influenced more
mainline medical publications and the potential positive benefits were accepted by subsequent mainline medical publications.[152]

Despite the taint of quackery, electrotherapeutics began to be considered a
justifiable part of medicine by the early twentieth century. It was often practiced in association with the new fields of radiology and radiation therapy.
Surgical applications of electroanesthesia were revived; it was even advocated
for major amputations.[153] Electricity was soon recognized as producing hypes-
thesia,[154] with experiments beginning in the 1920s and continuing today. Even
the Chinese eventually were drawn to electricity, which was incorporated as
part of the acupuncture process (electroacupuncture).

The mixture of legitimate practitioners and opportunists also persisted in
the twentieth century. For example, Albert Abrams claimed that a patient and
his or her organs were tuned to specific electromagnetic frequencies and

supplied devices with names such as the Dynamizer and Oscilloclast that, when tuned to the proper frequency, could diagnose and treat people, even at long distances. For his efforts, the American Medical Association ultimately named Dr. Abrams the Dean of Twentieth-Century Charlatans.[155]

Today, although mainstream medicine has employed techniques such as electrical cardioversion, cranial neuromagnetic stimulation, electroconvulsive therapy, and transcranial electrical nerve stimulation (TENS—albeit with contested results), its interests are not strongly focused on electromagnetic therapeutics. Still, the history of magnetism and electricity in medicine reveals a recurring pattern. An electric or magnetic therapy is first discovered, resisted by the medical establishment, and then discarded—only to arise again in the future in a slightly different form. The packaging and distribution of such devices has increased in sophistication but this pattern is likely to continue into the future until clear treatment benefits and a convincing mechanism of action are established.

ENERGY MEDICINE

The notion that living organisms possess some sort of special life force that gives them the unique quality called life is common in much of alternative medicine, but it has been a feature of the dominant medical practices throughout time. The belief in such a force appears to transcend cultures, called, in its various permutations, *prana* by the Hindus, *qi* by the Chinese, *ki* by the Japanese, and 95 other names in 95 other cultures.[156] This force is said to make up the source of life and is frequently associated with such concepts as soul, spirit, and mind. This belief is generally called *vitalism*. One succinct definition of the concept states that vitalism is "all the various doctrines which, from the time of Aristotle, have described things as actuated by some power or principle additional to mechanics and chemistry."[157]

In ancient times, the vital force was widely associated with breath. Breath was acknowledged to be a material substance and was described by the Greeks as *pneuma* and *psyche* and the Romans as *spiritus*. Words like *psychic* and *spirit* subsequently evolved to refer to nonmaterial and perhaps even supernatural qualities by which organisms are given life and consciousness.

While modern science was developing in the West, some scientists continued to look for scientific evidence for the nature of the force behind life. After Sir Isaac Newton published his classic laws of mechanics, optics, and gravity, he spent many years conducting alchemic experiments looking for the source of life. Given what was known in Newton's day, his gravity certainly had an occult quality to it—an invisible action being conducted at a distance. It was

---

"Energy Medicine" was written with Victor Stenger, PhD.

not unreasonable to consider that the forces of life had similar immaterial properties. Anton Mesmer's animal magnetism, discussed above, was simply another attempt to influence the unseen forces of life.

In the late nineteenth century, prominent scientists, including William Crooke and Oliver Lodge, sought scientific evidence for what they called the "psychic force," which they believed to be responsible for the mysterious powers of the mind. These powers were in full display in the popular mediums and spiritual charlatans of their day. Crooke and Lodge proposed that such thoughts might be connected with electromagnetic "aether waves."

As the nineteenth century drew to a close, experiments by Michelson and Morley had failed to find evidence for the aether. This laid the foundation for Einstein's theory of relativity and his photon theory of light, both published in 1905. The failure of the aether theory led to Max Planck's conjecture that light comes in bundles of energy called "quanta," thus triggering the quantum revolution. (These quanta are now recognized as material photons.)

The idea that matter alone can be responsible for life and the material body has never been popular. Modern veterinary medicine follows conventional biology, chemistry, and physics in treating the animal body as a complex, nonlinear system assembled from the same atoms and molecules that make up nonliving objects. In this sense, some aspects of veterinary medicine are very much like auto repair, in which broken parts in the animal machine get repaired or restored. Any look at veterinary technology reinforces this perception, what with devices to monitor blood pressure, heart rate, temperature, blood-oxygen content, and so on. For some, the "mechanics" of medicine is apparently unsatisfying.

As a result, and given the long-established history of vital energies in the human consciousness, it should come as no surprise that alternatives to such a mechanistic/naturalistic view become popular. For some with an alternative viewpoint, medicine can transcend the mere nuts and bolts, allowing treatment of what is considered to be the most important part of life—the vital force itself. Indeed, some people still consider that sentient beings possess a living field that may be linked to a deity, to the cosmos, or both. Life-force manipulations underlie acupuncture, chiropractic, homeopathy, and many other alternative approaches to medicine. A ready market exists for those who claim that they can succeed where medical science fails, or that their ministrations to the vital force can "complement" physiologically based therapies.

LASER AND LIGHT THERAPY

The concept that light, at intensities too low to heat or destroy tissue, can have biological effects has existed for centuries. Most ancient civilizations worshipped the sun or sun gods and appear to have made some connection between the light of the sun and health.[158] The ancient Greeks used sunlight to strengthen and heal. In ancient China, heliotherapy was one of the techniques employed by the early Daoists; a Tang dynasty (618–907 A.D.) ritual involved standing in the early morning, holding a piece of paper penned with the Chinese character for the sun, then shredding the paper in water and consuming it in an attempt to trap some of the sun's essence.[159]

The scientific foundations for the early practice of light therapy were not laid until the seventeenth and eighteenth centuries, beginning with observations by Sir Isaac Newton that sunlight could be refracted into its component parts by a prism (1666). The infrared and ultraviolet components of light were discovered at the turn of the nineteenth century by Sir Frederick Herschel in England and Johann Ritter in Germany. In 1877, Arthur Downes and Thomas Blunt showed that the ultraviolet (actinic) component of sunlight was lethal to bacteria and other microscopic organisms,[160] and this provided the impetus for the widespread use of phototherapy for the next 60 or 70 years. At the turn of the twentieth century, Nobel laureate Niels Finsen used red light to prevent the suppuration and scarring of patients who had contracted smallpox.[161] However, the gradual introduction of antibacterial agents in the twentieth century made phototherapy redundant in disease treatment. Still, as therapeutic uses of light waned, prophylactic uses rose, such as for rickets prevention, or simply for the maintenance of general health. Today, light certainly has diagnostic and therapeutic uses. For example, in medicine, ultraviolet radiation is used as a bactericide, in the treatment of psoriasis, and for the treatment of neonatal jaundice (unconjugated hyperbilirubinemia), and lasers have numerous applications in surgery.

Concurrent with the legitimate uses of ultraviolet phototherapy from the discoveries of Finsen until the mid-1950s was the rise of various quacks and charlatans. In 1876, Augustus Pleasonton, a retired Civil War general, published a blue book (with blue print) on the use of blue light for various ailments, including improving the growth of cattle.[162] John Harvey Kellogg, of breakfast cereal fame, devised various machines for the local and whole-body application of patients to visible light,[163] however, the machines contained simple incandescent light filaments that most likely caused thermal effects. Malaga, New Jersey, was home to the Spectrochrome Institute of Dinshah Ghaddiali, who infuriated the newly founded Food and Drug Administration with unfounded claims to have cured numerous diseases with his Spectro-Chrome instrument, which was simply a box containing a lightbulb, fitted with colored filters.[164] Various expensive types of light devices are currently marketed to animal owners, with a variety of diagnostic and therapeutic claims.[165] Some of these devices are simply made up of inexpensive light-emitting diodes (LEDs), others are diode lasers such as those used in laser pointers, and some are simply flashlights with colored tips.

A variant of phototherapy, laser therapy, was first used to treat humans in the late 1960s and early 1970s. These devices, with output powers of less than or equal to 1 mW are an extension of historical practice.[166] Laser therapy and light therapy owe much of their popularity to clinical trials and research begun in Hungary and the Eastern Bloc countries in the 1960s.[167,168] Reports that first filtered into the West were fragmentary and incomplete. Nevertheless, the work of these early investigators caught the attention of other researchers. Among the first effects reported were accelerated hair growth and wound healing, which early investigators believed to be due to laser or light stimulation of biological processes and the phenomenon was described as "biostimulation." However, it was later shown that low-intensity radiation could inhibit, as well as stimulate, cellular activity, and the term *biostimulation* has often been replaced or augmented with such terms as *low-intensity, low-power, low-level*, or *photon therapy*, terms that emphasize the nonthermal, low-energy characteristics of the approach. Today, low-power lasers are used in many parts of the world to treat musculoskeletal injury, pain, and inflammation.

Acceptance of this form of treatment is mixed. The U.S. Food and Drug Administration currently requires only a section 510K level of proof (that is, the devices must be substantially equivalent to other similar devices)[169] and low-power laser use is approved for neck pain, musculoskeletal pain, and the "pain associated with carpal tunnel syndrome." Still, the use by mainstream U.S. medical practitioners is limited, perhaps because the results of studies on the modality are equivocal. However, in Europe and other parts of the world, the situation is quite different. For example, low-power lasers were reported to be present in greater than 40 percent of physical therapy clinics in Great Britain and almost a third of Scandinavian dental clinics.[170]

The history of alternative medicine, indeed, of much of human history, is one of introduction of a new therapy or novel idea, curiosity and acceptance by an enthusiastic minority of practitioners and patients, skepticism by the part of the dominant medical authority, and gradual disuse of the new therapy as, ultimately, the claims of efficacy for the therapy fail to be demonstrated. Leaders of popular health "alternatives" have often attracted large followings, including people who are well educated. Alternative health movements can be thought of as ideologies that typically identify a few foundational aspects of health or healing, and often incorporate more universal feelings about people and nature, as well as the popular notions of individual eras.

Current claims for alternative approaches to veterinary medicine, be they for natural healing or against the purported harshness of mainstream therapies, are virtually identical to the claims that have been made for novel therapies in preceding centuries. In a few instances, effective therapies have emerged from unlikely or obscure beginnings and *have* ultimately shown their worth, in which case they have become subsumed into the medical mainstream. Overall, however, from a historical perspective, alternative medicine appears mostly to be a reflection of human nature in general, as seen in areas like fashion, where old styles disappear, to become new again after a wait of 20 or 30 years. It should be remembered that while it should be science based, medicine is also a human endeavor and subject to its foibles.

BIOGRAPHICAL NOTES

Paul D. Buell holds an MA in Chinese and a PhD in history and is an independent scholar, translator, and editor living in Seattle, Washington. He also works for Independent Learning, Western Washington University, in Bellingham. He is an adjunct professor of Western's Center for East Asian Studies, and the author of numerous books and articles, including his *Historical Dictionary of the Mongolian World Empire* (Lanham, MD, and Oxford: The Scarecrow Press, Inc. [Historical Dictionaries of Ancient Civilizations and Historical Eras, No. 8], 2003). He is an author-contributor for *Jane's Sentinel China and Northeast Asia*, and *Jane's Sentinel Russia and the CIS*.

Victor Stenger, holds a BS in electrical engineering from Newark College of Engineering, an MS in physics from UCLA, and a PhD in physics from UCLA. He was on the faculty of the University of Hawaii until 2000. He is currently Emeritus Professor of Physics and Astronomy at the University of Hawaii and Adjunct Professor of Philosophy at the University of Colorado. He has held visiting positions on the faculties of the University of Heidelberg in Germany, and Oxford in England, and has been a visiting researcher at Rutherford Laboratory in England, the National Nuclear Physics Laboratory in Frascati, Italy, and the University of Florence in Italy. Dr. Stenger's research career spanned the period of great progress in elementary particle physics that ultimately lead to the current standard model. He participated in experiments that helped establish the properties of strange particles, quarks, gluons, and neutrinos. He also helped pioneer the emerging fields of very high energy gamma ray and neutrino astronomy; his last experiment was a collaboration that showed that the neutrino has mass. He is the author of popular books that interface between physics, cosmology, philosophy, religion, and pseudoscience. These include *Not By Design: The Origin of the Universe* (1988); *Physics and Psychics: The Search for a World Beyond the Senses* (1990); *The Unconscious Quantum: Metaphysics in Modern Physics and Cosmology* (1995); *Timeless Reality: Symmetry, Simplicity, and Multiple Universes* (2000). His latest book is *Has Science Found God? The Latest Results in the Search for Purpose in the Universe* (2003)— all books by Prometheus Press, Amherst, NY. Much of his writing can be found at his website, http://spot.colorado.edu/~vstenger/.

Jeffrey Basford holds a PhD in experimental physics from the University of Minnesota and an MD from the University of Miami. He joined the Department of Physical Medicine and Rehabilitation at the Mayo Clinic, in Rochester, Minnesota, in 1982, where he is currently a professor of physical medicine and rehabilitation. His clinical interests are neurological rehabilitation and musculoskeletal pain. Dr. Basford has researched stroke and the physiologic effects of physical agents used in rehabilitative therapy on the human body. He has written chapters on physical agents for multiple physical medicine and rehabilitation textbooks in human medicine, and serves as the physician editor of *Archives of Physical Medicine and Rehabilitation.*

3

Science and Medical Therapy

THE NATURE OF SCIENTIFIC UNDERSTANDING OF THE WORLD

Many people appear not to think a great deal about the nature of knowledge. This may be true even for professionals, who may be too busy keeping up with current knowledge in immunology, hematology, quantum physics, or any number of other fields to worry about what is meant by knowledge, how knowledge is separated from belief, the ways in which knowledge claims can be validated, and so on. The general belief seems to be that knowledge is what is found in textbooks, reference books, and professional journals, and that is all that need be said.

The only time people are compelled to address questions about the nature of knowledge is when they face challenges from those who reject what the mainstream takes for granted. For example, a biologist may be put in such a position when a creationist rejects accepted knowledge about evolution, the age of the earth, or the fossil record. In the face of such challenges, it becomes natural to ask questions about how one's opponent validates claims about the age of the earth in a way other than use of carbon-14 dating or about the stability of species when confronted with the fossil record. Such debates are uncomfortable for experts because they usually involve confronting an opponent with radically different fundamental assumptions about what counts as knowledge—for example, the content of some sacred texts "literally interpreted," versus an objective measurement such as carbon dating. In such discussions, one is then *ipso facto* thrown into a philosophical discussion about the nature of knowledge of the world, or about the meaning of "literal interpretation," or about the very possibility of literal interpretation across different languages, and so on. It is often only in such contexts, challenging one's taken-for-granted views, that one is forced to get clear about one's own assumptions.

Most ordinary people and virtually all scientists accept empirical, evidence-based, scientific proof as the major modality for achieving knowledge of the physical world. This means that when they wish to understand something about the natural world—for example, why and how eclipses happen, how infectious diseases arise, what El Niño is and how it works—they reach for books and articles written by scientists or at least from a scientific point of view, not for books written by shamans, clergymen, theologians, or poets from a supernatural, mythic, literary, or divine justice point of view. Similarly, it means that when society wishes to research going to the moon, eliminating smallpox, waging a war against cancer, or increasing crop productivity, it awards grants to scientists at scientific research institutes, not to theosophists, projectors of astral bodies, or witch doctors.

The acceptance of science as the dominant way of knowing, first by intellectuals and eventually by society in general, is a fascinating and complex story, involving at various points philosophical revolutions, economic revolutions, as well as very practical considerations. For example, it is very likely that moving knowledge of the world into the purview of every man, rather than restricting it to the clergy and, to a lesser extent, to the aristocracy, is part and parcel of the move from monarchy to democracy, feudalism to capitalism, social rigidity to social mobility. For purposes of this book, however, it suffices to emphasize the relatively mundane reasons that science has solidly achieved supreme recognition in the Western social mind as the primary and undisputed modality for understanding the world, despite an extraordinary level of scientific illiteracy on the part of the general public, and despite a very nonscientific gullibility on the part of that population in a wide variety of areas, ranging from extraterrestrial visitations to receptivity to nonscientific medical alternatives. The reason science has become the predominant mode for accessing the world is, quite simply, that it *works*.

Most people, almost certainly today, have failed to distinguish between science and technology. For example, many people blame science for air pollution, environmental despoliation, unemployment, and other social ills that follow from major technological developments. And, indeed, at least since the industrial revolution, technology has been the public face of science, since relatively few members of the public care about science at a strictly theoretical, explanatory level. Nevertheless, science and technology, though intertwined, are distinct.

Even major critics of science, such as some animal rights advocates, nonetheless see science as unlimited in ability to understand and manipulate the empirical world. Perhaps paradoxically, one such advocate complained at a meeting that, since science could send a human to the moon, it could surely model a mouse on a computer and replace experimentation on animals! In a similar vein, the general public has no doubt that science will be able—and imminently—to genetically modify humans in whatever ways it chooses, or clone them, or cross human traits with animal traits. Indeed, it is not science as a way of knowing that the public ever doubts, rather, it is the motives, morality, and sanity of *scientists*, generating what has been termed *The Frankenstein Syndrome* regarding new technologies, particularly biological ones.[1] If there is skepticism about science, it is not about its ability to penetrate and manipulate nature's secrets. It is far more about whether such a powerful tool should be placed in the hands of scientists who seem to ignore the ethical and prudential implications of new technology!

In any case, science as a way of knowing has become solidly established as *the* way of knowing in the eyes of society. For many people, educated and less-educated alike, it is difficult to imagine any other approach to knowing about the world—and effecting change in the world by predicting and controlling what happens—besides science. The very word *science* has indeed become synonymous with any sort of knowing at all. The word is even used to garner credibility for certain fields. For example, people talk of library science, consumer science, and so on, even if these fields are not sciences in any clear sense.

This in turn suggests the futility of seeking an algorithmic "scientific method" that obtains across all empirical disciplines. Obviously the methodology used to test hypotheses in chemistry is very different from the methodology used to test hypotheses in particle physics (where the entities discussed are not directly observable), which is very different from the methodology used to test social science hypotheses or linguistic ones or ethological ones or evolutionary ones or cosmological ones. But there are certain key notions that characterize a scientific approach to testing any hypothesis.

Reason—At its root, science is based in reason and logic. Logical inconsistency, incoherence, and other obvious forms of irrationality are to be filtered out of scientific discourse. (There are historical exceptions, such as the interpretation of quantum mechanics that suggests that quantum phenomena violate the law of noncontradiction.)

Replicability—Science is committed to the principle of uniformity of nature, that is, that under similar circumstances, like causes produce like effects. Another way to make this point is that science sees the world as rule-governed, and phenomena as exhibiting regularities or laws. This implies that any experimental result should be repeatable by recreating the circumstances of the experiment. The famous cases of alleged psychic powers that move physical objects or the alleged achievement of cold fusion are instances where reported results are rejected for lack of replicability, among other reasons.

Removal of Observer or Experimenter Bias—This is related to the previous notion. There are numerous cases in the history of science of researcher expectation (such as the Rosenthal effect),* theoretical commitments, vested interest, and so on influencing experimental results, as in Gregor Mendel's data or Einstein's jocular remark that had Eddington's data not confirmed the general theory of relativity, "so much the worse for the data." Scientific practice has worked to minimize this corruptive influence by developing an extensive field of experimental design, statistical methods for power of experiments, repeatability criteria, blind and double-blind protocols, all intended to suppress bias in experimentation. From a philosophical point of view, scientific thinking is based on certain assumptions. Generally scientists assume that there is an objective world out there existing independently of perception. (Interestingly enough, this is a philosophical assumption, in that it cannot be proven empirically.) At the same time, people's only access to the world is through inherently subjective perceptions, which are notoriously subject to error and bias and wishful thinking. The methods and rules of experimental science have been developed under the assumption that people can access the objective world by careful control and monitoring, by summing subjective perceptions gathered according to experimental rules. Individual perception is fallible, but collective perceptions gathered according to rules of scientific inquiry generate collectively an objective reality.

Prediction and Control—Given the previous commitments, it follows that science should give people the power to predict events in the world, and within the limits of technological capability, control or alter them. (Note that prediction also includes what has been called "retrodiction," predicting backward, as when we use our knowledge of natural regularities to explain what has already occurred. In science, predicting the future and explaining the past are symmetrical.) It is for this reason that scientists are suspicious of theoretical endeavors such as psychoanalysis, where few psychoanalysts can generate predictions about an individual human's behavior, although they are quite willing to explain past behavior. For example,

---

*The tendency for results to conform to experimenters' expectations unless stringent safeguards are instituted to minimize bias; named after Robert Rosenthal, who did many of the original experiments showing the problem.

whereas a psychoanalyst might explain Hitler's obsession with exterminating Jews by appeal to his early toilet training, he or she would never predict that someone toilet trained the same way today would grow up obsessed with exterminating Jews. Ability to retrodict but not predict is often seen by scientists as the mark of pseudosciences like astrology, though such problems also plague social science and evolutionary biology.

Reductionism—The notion that the best science is the science that most completely embodies the foregoing principles obviously follows from these principles. The best science is in turn believed to be mechanistic physics and chemistry, where the laws are most completely described, where it is most possible to predict and control, and where people can best generate controlled experimentation. This is neatly evidenced by the inexorable ascendance in status (and funding) of molecular biology over organismic biology. In general, this view affirms that we have the most complete explanations when we have expressed the phenomenon to be explained in terms of physical and chemical reactions. In its extreme form, as expressed by some logical positivists, this view says that human psychology, history, and sociology can be explained by reducing human behavior to neurophysiology and thence to physicochemistry. Part and parcel of reductionism is the dismissal of anything not clearly reducible to physicochemistry from the purview of "real science," including things such as subjective states and value judgments, untestable notions like life force, absolute space and time, and other such notions that had crept into science, as well as for all philosophical claims not subject to empirical test.

Thus, the twentieth century saw psychology methodologically eschew talk about mental states and transform itself into the study of overt behavior in the movement known as behaviorism. It is not surprising that, in the face of what we have discussed, behaviorism was sold to the public as a movement turning psychology into real science, with an attendant technology of behavior allowing us to shape human behavior (e.g., away from criminality). Accordingly, for most of the twentieth century, talk of subjective states became scientifically anathema.[2]

In the same spirit, science began to trumpet itself as value-free, in general, and ethics-free, in particular. Whether one looks at the responses of atomic scientists to queries about work on the atomic bomb or examines textbooks of biology as late as 1990, one finds scientists disavowing an obligation to deal with ethical issues, claiming instead that ethics is the task of society, not science.

If one looks at the history of science, one finds an inexorable tendency for the sciences to fit themselves into the just-defined template. Beginning with astronomy and physics, moving to chemistry and biology and eventually to psychology, linguistics, and social science, studies of various aspects of the world have struggled to fit into the criteria just delineated. In doing so, they have ruthlessly expunged from their purview anything perceived as failing to fit those criteria. (A classic and not-so-surprising account of the zealous application of the above can be found in Francis Crick's *Of Molecules and Men*,[3] from the scientist who effected perhaps the most important step in moving biology into physicochemistry.)

MEDICINE AND SCIENCE

Relative to its history, medicine has not long been under the influence of the science model. One event often credited with marking the transition to a science-based medicine (probably exaggeratedly, since the relevant changes had already begun) is the 1910 publication of the *Flexner Report*, by Abraham Flexner,[4] an educator who attacked medical education's failing to reflect the increase in scientific knowledge, and most medical schools as grossly inadequate. (No less a literary luminary than Mark Twain regularly attacked "orthodox" medical therapies as unproven and even harmful.) Flexner further argued that rather than being entrepreneurial activities, medical schools should be attached to universities so as to benefit from the development of science relevant to medicine. Flexner's report gave further impetus to a movement toward incorporating science into medicine that had been fueled by the founding in 1903 of the Rockefeller Institute for Medical Research and with the American Medical Association's promoting of science as a basis for medicine.

Until well after the Flexner Report, mainstream medicine was as empirically useless, and even harmful, as were the dozens of competitors it had, from snake oil to hydrotherapy to herbalism to homeopathy. There was little difference in validation between the mainstream use of bleeding, mercury, quinine, salts, and other useless and harmful therapies and the ministrations of alternative competitive therapies. Mark Twain, in fact, lampooned the many patients who combined *all* available therapeutic modalities, saying, "Then there were those who saw good in everything and who believed that whatever is, is right, and these last mixed the allopathic, homeopathic, and hydropathic systems, qualified each with each, and thus passed to their homes, drenched, pickled, sweetened and soaked"[5] (perhaps foreshadowing the attitudes of those drawn to "complementary" treatments today). By the 1930s, human medicine was pretty well subordinated to the science-based medical model and has continued to grow exponentially in the same direction.

Veterinary medicine has followed more or less the same pathway as human medicine, albeit more slowly and haltingly, given the relative differences in funding support. The National Institutes of Health began funding veterinary schools and researchers therein in the late 1950s. By the 1970s, the Colorado

State University veterinary school was comfortable enough with this model to change its name from the College of Veterinary Medicine to the College of Veterinary Medicine and Biomedical Sciences. The research and curricula one finds in medical and veterinary schools are very similar—indeed curriculum for the first two years of medical school is virtually the same for human and animal medicine. With the subordination of veterinary medicine to the science model, the social credibility of veterinary medicine has increased, and the somewhat derogatory "horse doctor" image has been replaced by something closer to that of a physician, though without much of the "baggage" physicians carry (veterinarians enjoy greater credibility). When the American Veterinary Medical Association assumed responsibility for accrediting veterinary colleges, the science model was further solidified, since solidity in the basic sciences is a *sine qua non* for accreditation.

At any rate, it is fair to say that, by the mid–twentieth century, all of medicine, human and veterinary, had become science based, at least in principle, and, as the century continued, the science base was increasingly solidified in fact. In particular, the development of drug therapies by the scientific methods of testing and validation provided a powerful armamentarium against disease, unprecedented in the history of civilization. Great optimism about the future of medicine prevailed; diseases like smallpox were eradicated, and life expectancies for humans and companion animals were extended.

In light of these accomplishments, it is fair to ask, why has there been an ever-increasing dissatisfaction with science-based medicine since the 1960s? As an even more important corollary, why have some citizens in society as well as some physicians and veterinarians been drawn to non-science-based alternative medical approaches—chiropractic, homeopathy, herbalism, aroma therapy, colored lights, acupuncture, magnet therapy, electro-therapy, and the like?

REASONS FOR DISAFFECTION WITH THE SCIENCE MODEL

There are many reasons for the development in society of a yearning for another sort of medicine. This has, in turn, led to people uncritically embracing alternative therapies.

In addition to providing a way of knowing, science also provides a worldview, or a metaphysic. To take a simple example, if one adopts the view that the world is all and only what science tells us it is, a view that many scientists hold—although others do not—one cannot also logically believe in God, a plan to the world, divine punishment, disembodied spirits, Heaven, and so on. Such entities are excluded by the demand for empirical verification of what we claim to exist. Direct evidence for any of the above is unavailable, and in any case, it is difficult to say what might count as acceptable evidence. This is in contradistinction to testing for the existence of unicorns, a case in which what would constitute acceptable evidence would be generally agreed upon.

However, science may encounter two difficulties when it comes to resolving real-world debates. First, science cannot absolutely prove a universal judgment, as David Hume powerfully demonstrated in the eighteenth century. That is, no matter how well a theory or observation is established, it is always at least *theoretically* possible that some new bit of information will come along to overturn previous observations. For example, although the laws of gravity appear to be universal, there *might* be some previously unknown location at which those laws are suspended, where one might rise up into the air if one were to come across it on a hike. Science cannot prove that such a place doesn't exist, but as time passes, and such places fail to come to light, the certitude in which the laws of gravity are held increases. However, the mere fact that such unlikely possibilities *might* exist does not also serve as a reason to hold out hope that they will be discovered, nor can therapeutic approaches be legitimately based on such speculation.

The second difficulty of science is that it cannot be used to resolve debates where evidence does not exist, or in situations where what constitutes acceptable evidence cannot be agreed upon. So, for example, what might constitute acceptable evidence for the existence of a Heaven, or a God, would likely vary greatly among individuals. In addition, such evidence is clearly not important insofar as establishing beliefs in such concepts, which are not encompassed in the worldview of science. However, when the worldview implicit in science clashes with a personal worldview based on belief, a reason to doubt the validity of science may be created (instead of the other way around).

This is especially true and personal when it comes to scientific medicine. For example, one major metaphysical or reality clash between ordinary common sense and science concerns the perceived uniqueness of the individual. In reductionist science, no individual is special, that is, the same universal laws apply to everyone. One carbon molecule or electron or HIV particle or chemical reaction of a certain sort or falling body of a certain mass is indistinguishable from any other. Unfortunately, for some, this results in a depersonalization of the entire medical transaction. Indeed, concentrating on the process, rather than the individual, some physicians or veterinarians may have spoken of "the kidney in Room 103," "the patent ductus arteriosis," or "the mammary tumor," rather than "Mary Jones" or "Fred Smith" or "Spot." Individuality and personhood in such cases may have been subordinated to the universal, lawlike, and repeatable. As such, physicians may have been perceived as treating instances of diseases, not unique persons.

This gestalt represented a major shift from that of pre-science-based medicine, wherein medicine was seen as an art, or a combination of art and science. Traditionally, as far back as Aristotle, art deals with the unique, with the individual as individual, whereas science deals with the universal, with the individual as an instance of a law or generality. Sick people and owners of sick animals, particularly companion animals, do not see themselves or their animals as replaceable, interchangeable instances of a scientific universal. They all feel well or sick, that they are unique, and that their sicknesses are *theirs*, not that they *are* the sicknesses! Insofar as scientifically oriented physicians and veterinarians failed to recognize, as Oliver Sacks argued in *Awakenings*,[6] that a disease is always a unique complex of individuality and universality, they risked losing credibility with ordinary people to whom one's uniqueness, and the uniqueness of one's disease, was a nonnegotiable fact.

This is not merely abstract metaphysical conflict. Insofar as science-based medical practitioners ignore the individuality of a patient, they may tend to lack empathy—"this is just another . . ." How else can the countless stories of practitioner (especially specialist) callousness—oncologists telling patients that if they have problems with radiation or chemotherapy, call the nurse; physicians and veterinarians coolly informing a patient or client that "you," "your animal," or "your mother" has one month to live—be explained? Indeed, given scientific medical and veterinary specialization and the time demands on practitioners, the all-too-frequently short amount of contact between patients and their doctors militates against any relationship being formed, and further reinforces the idea of sickness as repeatable instances of a universal, the idea of care as an abstraction.

This, in turn, may lead people to seek help and solace elsewhere. Suppose a person has a dog with a tumor. He or she travels 60 miles to an oncologist at a veterinary school. The oncologist examines the animal, performs tests, and comes back with a diagnosis of metastatic adenocarcinoma. He then tells the owner that the dog is basically doomed and suggests they think about euthanasia when symptoms warrant it. Scientifically sound, quick and dirty, over and done with. Nevertheless, and in spite of the facts, this may be difficult to accept for the client, both emotionally and psychologically. Say then that a neighbor tells the client of an herbalist (or light therapist or whatever) who supposedly helped another dog with cancer. The client goes to the herbalist. The herbalist guarantees nothing, but is very, very understanding, talks to the client about the dog for a full half hour, asks about the client-animal relationship, pets the dog, and promises to do his or her absolute best.

While not necessarily supplying effective therapy, the herbalist does supply something the oncologist does not—comfort for the client, empathy, conversation, hope, and recognition of individuality and uniqueness. These are part of the client's view of medicine, albeit not the oncologist's. The end, of course, is the same. Yet it is very likely that the client will say that the herbalist is an excellent doctor and the oncologist is not.

In the end, what do most clients and patients mean by "excellent doctor"? They mean that they received solace and empathy and concern and conversation, not necessarily that anyone was cured. (It is well known that 70–90 percent of acute diseases are self-limiting, and it has been estimated in human medicine that of some fifty thousand medical conditions, cures exist for only about two thousand.) Thus, if doctors approach patients or clients as repeated instances of similar pathophysiology and fail to understand the psychological dynamic of the doctor-patient (or, in veterinary medicine, doctor-client) interaction, this may fuel, at least in some people, a search for alternatives.

A second reason that some people have embraced alternative medicine flows from what has been previously discussed, that is, scientific medicine's ideological tendency to deny the reality and/or knowability of subjective states—thoughts, feelings, emotions, and so on—since these states are not observable or quantifiable or objectively measurable. Physicians and veterinarians have, for most of the twentieth century, been uncomfortable talking about notions like quality of life, subjective pain, and suffering, all notions that are difficult and perhaps impossible to quantify. For example, one can find virtually no literature on suffering in human and veterinary medicine—nor even a medical dictionary definition! As a result, pain, suffering, fear, distress, and quality of life (among others) may have been set aside by scientific medical practitioners as at least medically irrelevant, if not unreal.

As one nursing dean once wisely said, "Physicians worry only about *cure*. We (nurses) worry about *care*." In veterinary medicine, an extraordinary series of papers powerfully demonstrated the degree to which veterinary medicine has ignored patient comfort.[7,8,9,10] For physicians, a victory over disease is keeping the patient alive longer—that is a measurable win. That the longer life is at the expense of suffering, family stress, or patient dignity has historically not been the concern of the scientific specialist. In the United States, heroic centers for veterinary oncology are flourishing, and animals may be kept alive after multiple limb amputations and mandiblectomies, with little apparent regard for the animal's quality of life.

This situation is paralleled in human medicine, where a widespread and somewhat cavalier disregard for pain appears to exist, especially in such fields as oncology and orthopedics. Physicians have opposed marijuana and morphine for terminally ill suffering patients out of fear of addiction. Daniel Callahan[11] and others,[12] have argued that if physicians paid more attention to how patients feel, there would be less furor over assisted suicide and euthanasia—patients fear pain and suffering, and that is why they want to die. Correlatively, it has been reported that although 90 percent of cancer pain is controllable, 80 percent of it is not controlled. And the situation is even worse in pediatrics where, until 1990, open-heart surgery on infants was done with paralytic drugs, not anesthetics and analgesics, on the grounds that the latter two were dangerous. This sort of behavior is in turn buttressed by the definition of pain adopted by the International Society for the Study of Pain, which affirms that the possession of language is a necessary condition for being able to feel pain.[13]

Veterinary medicine, too, was—some would say still is—enormously delinquent about pain,[14] with many procedures done with "bruticaine" (brute force) or paralytics, and virtually no literature on animal analgesia until federal laboratory animal law compelled the growth of use and research into animal analgesia. There were (and still are), in fact, a host of rationalizations widespread among veterinarians to support not worrying about the pain that animals feel. To wit:

- Many veterinarians still call anesthesia "sedation" or "chemical restraint."
- One may hear that anesthesia is "more stressful than the surgical procedure performed without anesthesia."
- Postsurgical analgesics are not needed because animals will "eat immediately after surgery."
- Analgesics are not to be used because without the pain, the animal will inexorably reinjure the damaged body part.
- Postsurgical howling and whining are not signs of pain, they are "after-effects of anesthesia."
- Anatomical differences, such as the presence of an anatomical mesenteric sling, vitiate the need for pain control after abdominal surgery in the dog.
- Animals do not need postsurgical analgesia because we can watch them behave normally after surgery.
- Young animals feel less pain than older ones, and thus do not need surgical anesthesia for procedures like tail-docking or castration.
- Analgesia deadens the coping ability of predators, and thus is more discomfiting to an animal than the pain is.
- Liver biopsies don't hurt.

And so on.

Though there are adequate—even definitive—responses to all of these spurious reasons, they persist as barriers against pain management. Indeed, as one drug company executive has said, by their reckoning, approximately one-third of veterinarians don't use analgesia. This is buttressed by a statement made by the executive director of one large state veterinary association who expressed amazement that so many veterinarians fail to supply pain control despite the fact that it is easy and lucrative, and causes remarkable positive changes in the animal's demeanor. Finally, many veterinarians do not know a great deal about pain management. In a 1996 paper, Dohoo and Dohoo showed that veterinarians' knowledge in the field of pain management is quite limited, and that what practitioners do know is typically not acquired in veterinary school.[15]

Although to the scientifically minded human medical or veterinary practitioner, pain may seem to be a relatively unimportant side effect of disease or injury, we now in fact know that pain is a biologically active stressor that can increase the likelihood of infection, retard wound healing, create immunosuppression, and even promote metastasis of malignant neoplasms. Even more important, to the patient or client, pain is *everything*. And the animal in pain may even be worse off than the human in pain because, as Ralph Kitchell has remarked, the animal cannot, as humans do, anticipate an end to the pain, and thus has no hope.[16]

If a physician or veterinarian gives short shrift to a person's or an animal's pain—indeed, to any condition—the patient or client will naturally gravitate elsewhere, however implausible the elsewhere may be. This is particularly true in society today, where the notion of pain tolerance as a badge of character has all but disappeared, except perhaps among athletes. Indeed, eliminating any sort of discomfort seems to be a current social obsession. And veterinary clients, of course, extend this to their animals.

Thus, as in the previous discussion of individuality, when scientific medicine ignored or devalued or bracketed felt pain, it dealt itself a serious blow, since people sought alleviation of and sympathy for their pain elsewhere. And many alternative therapists are *exceedingly* sympathetic and empathetic, thereby in some sense making people feel better even though they did little about pain based in organic-somatic causes. In fact, they may have even helped the cause of pain if it were psychogenic, or perhaps even chronic. Such cases elude pharmacological management and, in many cases, both in people and in animals, such conditions may be best handled through deflection of attention from it. But the key point is that alternative therapies provided something people may not have been getting from scientific human and veterinary medicine.

A third reason for the rise of alternative therapies is sociocultural and has to do with what might be called a "new openness" in society or, depending on one's philosophy, a "new softheadedness," beginning in the 1960s. Prior to the 1960s, people were quite comfortable in their xenophobia and ethnocentrism. Subsequently, hippies and counterculturals effectively wiped the slate clean, and respect for other cultures became *de rigueur*. In particular, Eastern cultures and primitive cultures (a sort of neo-eighteenth-century noble-savage view) were held in high esteem. In many cases, the cultures respected were little understood or misunderstood, but that didn't matter. For example, the Jains are much touted for the extraordinary lengths to which they go not to kill even insects, and are seen as humane exemplars. Perhaps paradoxically, they will not euthanize an animal however much it is suffering; their concern for animal life stems from the religious idea that animals are reincarnated humans, not out of primary concern for the animal's welfare.

Certainly, there are long-established traditions of other cultures, some of it quite sophisticated. Chinese medicine has a very long and documented history (albeit generally misunderstood or misinterpreted). Doctors in India performed surgeries such as cataract removal thousands of years ago. Further respecting the observations of long-established cultures, the drug companies—no hippies, to be sure—have for decades employed ethnopharmacologists seeking plants and herbs and animal products used by primitive societies for medicaments. So it is perfectly rational and legitimate and sensible to look to other cultures for clues regarding therapeutic agents and approaches.

Still, there is much difference between curiosity and respect and uncritical acceptance. For example, drug companies do not merely harvest traditional plants and package them for customers. Instead, they will scientifically test therapeutic candidates for safety and efficacy under controlled conditions using standardized experimental protocols. Unfortunately, many people in society skip the validation part and simply assume that something works just because it comes from another culture.

In addition, since the 1960s, society has exhibited an occultistic, mystical tendency, which prompted one Catholic priest to say that despite the "Godlessness" of the 1960s, the mind-set developed then contained so much religious orientation that it would eventually bring people back to the Church, which was well equipped to meet spiritual needs. This is evidenced by resurgent social interest in astrology, crystals, magic, witchcraft (or wicca), out-of-body experiences, extraterrestrial visitation, cults, angels, and other areas actively sneered at and dismissed by science. At any rate, such a mind-set again favored the move toward alternative medicines, especially when it was cloaked in spiritual or holistic raiment.

Finally, since the 1960s, many members of society have criticized science-based medicine as being too oriented toward cure and therapy for disease, and not sufficiently focused on prevention, wellness, lifestyle, nutrition, and so on. This in turn draws people toward alternative traditions that allegedly focus on healthy ways of living.

There are likely a host of other reasons why some members of society have embraced alternative medicine. However, the real issue is, what is the appropriate response of science-based medicine to these challenges? This is the issue that must be addressed.

BABIES AND BATH WATER

Many of the concerns that have been previously enumerated and that have driven people to alternative medicine are legitimate and need to be taken seriously by scientific medicine. Unfortunately, scientific medicine has been caught up in what has been called scientific ideology, that is, the set of assumptions that is uncritically taught to nascent scientists along with the empirical facts of their respective disciplines. These include the infamous notion that science is "value free" and doesn't make ethical judgments. The result is that science has allowed others to define the social and ethical issues emerging from scientific advances and, as the issues of genetic engineering and cloning demonstrate, has been constantly on the defensive.

In any case, legitimate criticisms of science-based medicine following from what we have discussed include but are not necessarily limited to the following:

- Insufficient concern for the patient as individual.
- Insufficient attention to pain, suffering, and other subjective states.
- Insufficient attention paid to social-ethical concerns about medicine.
- Insufficient attention paid to public literacy about scientific and medical advances.
- Insufficient attention paid to educating the public vis-à-vis scientific validation of therapies, medicaments, and so on.
- Insufficient attention to the medical traditions of other cultures as a possible source of therapies.
- Insufficient attention to preventive medicine and maintenance of health rather than curing disease.
- Insufficient attention to side effects of drugs and other therapies, which can devastate one's life.

Many of these deficiencies are being remedied, but even if they were not, one overwhelming logical point must be kept in mind. *Nothing in what has been previously discussed casts one iota of doubt on basing acceptance or rejection of therapeutic modalities upon evidence-based controlled experimentation.* Even if every single criticism of science-based medicine reflected in social yearning for alternatives were correct, nothing in these criticisms favors any other method of proof for therapies. The proof of a therapy is whether it can be demonstrated to work—to be effective. If there is agreement upon methods for testing therapies, they should be equally applied to all therapeutic candidates.

While a small minority of alternative practitioners may suggest that the tools of science cannot be applied to their particular therapies (for example, homeopaths may suggest that their individualized therapies cannot be subjected to randomized, controlled clinical trials), most people, including the U.S. government-funded National Center for Complementary and Alternative Medicine, disagree.[17] At best, proponents of alternative medical approaches have raised suggestions about possible alternative sources of therapies, changes in emphasis in medical research, even changes in the values underlying medicine. But no one has pointed out flaws in the way in which scientific medicine does validate the therapies it considers, or has suggested new methods of validation. (Indeed, some advocates of alternative therapies press for scientific validation of therapeutic candidates and fault science-based medicine mainly for ignoring plausible sources for therapies.) In fact, if one is interested in undercutting evidence-based, controlled experimental protocols for testing therapies for safety and efficacy, attacking the logical basis of experimental design, a methodology designed to go beyond unfounded or uncorroborated subjective feelings, is the only way to accomplish it.

SCIENTIFIC TESTING AND ITS ALTERNATIVES

Consider the common *post hoc ergo propter hoc* fallacy of logic ("after this therefore because of this"). A remedy is applied–the condition improves. Is it therefore warranted to conclude that the remedy was responsible for the improvement? Certainly not: the correlation might be entirely coincidental. The effect (improvement) might have occurred even if the alleged cause did not occur; the effect might even have been caused by something other than the suggested cause. How does one distinguish between real causes and effects and temporal associations?

Controlled experimentation allows people to answer such questions by comparing treatments by use of groups receiving an experimental treatment, and eliminates subjective bias by use of such things as double-blind and randomized protocols. Have those who advocate untested therapies found logical flaws in such methodology? No. Have such advocates suggested a different and better way to test therapies and explained this new methodology? No. Is there a method for distinguishing effective from ineffective therapies implicit or explicit in the writings of those who advocate alternatives? There are none that have become apparent.

Thus, the advocacy for alternative therapies ends in one of two possible conclusions. Such advocates may say that we should cast a wider net in searching for new therapies but reserve judgment about safety and efficacy of any new therapeutic candidates, whatever their source, until we test them. Such a stance would seem to be inarguable–indeed, the scientific methodology is the essence of open-mindedness and fairness. It is an obvious truism, analogous to saying that college admissions officers should look beyond wealthy private schools for candidates that meet admission standards. On the other hand, if advocates are saying that some therapies do not need testing, or are in some way self-validating, or that there are better standards for testing than those that are currently in use, they are obliged to say why these therapies need no testing or to specify the better standards for testing, and why and how they are better. Not doing so is like saying college admissions officers should admit certain students who do not meet admission standards, but failing to specify the reasons. Otherwise stated, there is every reason to look in new places for therapies, but there is no good reason to drop the standards of proof.

The bars that have been set up to test efficacy and safety are not arbitrary principles of etiquette and style; they are the result of hundreds of years of logical refinement aimed at eliminating unfounded claims, subjective bias, misidentification of cause and effect, and so on. The most damaging thing one can say of these standards is that sometimes they are circumvented, for extralogical reasons. Scientists may falsify data and drug companies may conceal damaging data; as a result, journals and conferences now ask for conflict of interest information. Indeed, mainstream science-based medicine may use treatments that have not been tested by proper methods. But such abuses do not indict or even call these standards into question, any more than Hitler's rantings cast doubt on the validity of logic, or a ministerial sex scandal invalidates the tenets of Christianity to its followers.

However, using just such reasoning, many alternative medicine advocates claim that since science-based medicine uses many unproven therapies their own unproven practices are justified. At best this is a *tu quoque* ("you, too") fallacy. If you are accused of reasoning fallaciously in a certain case, it is no defense for you to point out an occasion where the accuser had done the same thing. Furthermore, the extent to which unproven therapies are employed in human medicine appears to have been greatly exaggerated.[18]

Ultimately, having the issue at hand as a debate over alternative or complementary therapies obscures the real issue. What is really at stake is the difference between validated and nonvalidated therapy. When a therapy—any therapy—can meet accepted standards, it is no longer an alternative. It is proven. Any therapy that fails to meet these standards is simply unproven and, to the extent that it eschews them, unscientific. What is truly alternative has more to do with historical accident (i.e., when something is tested) than it has to do with logic.

SUMMARY

In summary, science is the socially dominant modality for knowing about the world. The features that make up a science-based approach to validation of a hypothesis of any sort have been described. Medicine, human and veterinary, became science based in the twentieth century. When medicine became science based, it tended to emphasize regularities and de-emphasize individuality, and also tended to de-emphasize judgments of quality of life and subjective states of pain and suffering. This, in turn, led to some social disaffection with science-based medicine, and to a social movement embracing alternative therapies. However valid the social criticism was of science-based medicine in the above areas, these criticisms are totally irrelevant to how one can judge empirical claims, including therapeutic claims of safety and efficacy. Insofar as science is the only socially accepted method of validating such claims, therapies are either validated scientifically or not at all, since no one has argued for alternative methods of validation.

The question that remains to be asked is this: could society (and medical professionals) choose to reject a science-based, socially sanctioned approach to medicine in favor of something else? What would that something else look like? What are the arguments for and against such an approach? And what effect would this have on veterinary and human medicine? These questions will be engaged in the ensuing chapters.

4

Ethics, Evidence, and Medicine

The lure of alternative, or non-evidence-based, medicine is undeniable, and the temptation to succumb to it can be irresistible. Based on enthusiastic promotions read during periods when one's energy flags, one might pop ginseng, chug awful-tasting but expensive tonics, or align one's bed with the earth's electrical impulses or Feng-Shui lines! Do such things work? Who knows? How can such things be tested? If, after doing such things, people feel more energetic, how can they know that they were not experiencing wishful thinking, or falling victim to observer bias, in the well-known manner of the Rosenthal effect or Dumbo's feather? Nonetheless, people continue to succumb to such temptations thinking, "What harm does it do?" or "Stranger things have happened!"

People are not so civilized or sophisticated that they have lost the lifeline to magic thinking: witness perennial fascination with alien abductions, yeti, and the Bermuda Triangle. In their nonprofessional moments, that is, most of the time, scientists are as vulnerable to the lure of the non–science based as anyone else. For example, professionals in the biological sciences may also be creationists in their private lives; reductionist physicists and philosophers may be very Aristotelian in their daily lives.

This point was brought home very dramatically on a committee established at a major university to award small "seed money" grants to worthy researchers. All the other committee members were senior scientists, with the exception of a token humanist representing the College of Liberal Arts, needed to meet a legal requirement. Twice a year, the committee members would meet and receive their assignments of submitted protocols, which would then be reviewed for a month, prior to reconvening to make the awards.

The committee appeared not to know what to do with the humanist. Finally, he was given two protocols, one on mycorhyzoids, as mycorhyzoids are important for food production, food production is an ethical issue, and the humanist was a philosopher. The other protocol pertained to music therapy, which was the only submission from the College of Liberal Arts. The humanist, concerned that he might disgrace himself, or his field, spent an inordinate amount of time mastering the scientific protocols. Subsequently, when it was time for the committee to discuss the music therapy protocol, which involved a request to fund an organ to try to teach autistic children to speak, the humanist was very critical of it, as no evidence had been cited to support any connection between organ music and acquisition of language, not even a reasonable hypothesis regarding a connection. In the humanist's view, the researcher simply wanted money for an organ! The objections were articulated; the humanist's conclusions were that the proposal, even though it came from the humanist's college, was neither conceptually nor empirically well founded and should not be funded.

Shockingly, the committee chairman looked directly into the humanist's eyes and intoned, "Well I don't know about you, but I for one want to leave no stone unturned to try to help those poor children, and I'm surprised you don't." Worse still, all the other members were nodding and looking disapprovingly at the humanist, as if he were Scrooge. The rest of the committee unanimously voted to fund the project. The humanist's rejoinder of "Why don't you hire a witch doctor?" was ignored. *Mirabile dictu*, all but one member of the committee were accomplished scientists!

Everyone, and particularly those whose vocation is healing, wants to help the afflicted. So it is understandable that those people are drawn to untested modalities and alternative modalities sanctified by public demand and by anecdotal testimonials. After all, where is the harm? In fact, there is indeed considerable ethical mischief in such an attitude. In fact every major ethical vector relevant to veterinary medicine is actually or potentially compromised by failing to hold to a demand for a scientific evidentiary base for treatment modalities.

Other writings have outlined the sorts of ethical vectors confronting veterinarians and creating the complex skein that is veterinary ethics.[1] Veterinarians, like physicians, have obligations to clients, society, peers, and their profession, and to themselves. What makes veterinary ethics in some ways more difficult and complex than human medical ethics is that veterinarians also have an obligation to their patients, the animals, who are not the same as their clients. Unlike the case of pediatricians, society is relatively silent about codifying our moral obligations to those patients. Accordingly, non-evidence-based medicine—be it accepted or alternative—must be examined in terms of the moral categories relevant to veterinary decision making.

SOCIETAL OBLIGATIONS

Veterinarians, like other professionals, have obligations to society in general. Society grants professionals special privileges (such as writing prescriptions and doing surgery) in virtue of the function they are expected to perform. In addition, society gives a considerable degree of autonomy to professionals and is loath to regulate professions to any considerable extent, since legislators lack the requisite familiarity with the nature of veterinary practice. Instead, society, in essence, says to veterinarians, "You regulate yourselves the way we would regulate you if we understood in detail what you do (which we don't), but if you violate this charge and trust we will know and hammer you with Draconian rules."

A good example of this can be found some years ago. At that time, it became clear that some veterinarians were overprescribing antibiotics for growth promotion in livestock and thereby also promoting the development of antibiotic-resistant pathogens. This, in turn, created a danger to human health. Congress reacted by considering legislation that would have eliminated extra-label drug use for veterinarians, a move that would, in essence, have hamstrung veterinary medicine. This example clearly demonstrates that if veterinary medicine wishes to preserve its autonomy, it has a prudential as well as moral reason to respect society's demands and conditions.

In any event, it is evident that among society's expectations of veterinarians (and, for that matter, of all medical professionals) is one that they be solidly rooted in science and a scientific approach. This is clearly illustrated in myriad ways. The first line of the veterinary oath commits a veterinarian "to use my *scientific knowledge* [emphasis added] and skills for the benefit of society." Again, presuppositional to the accreditation of veterinary schools (graduation from which is in turn presuppositional to licensure) is instruction in *biomedical sciences*, as well as "substantial research activities" in the sciences. And, whereas the defense against malpractice used to be consonance with the practices of one's peers, more and more one must refer to veterinary textbooks, which are science based.

In other words, veterinary practitioners are chartered by society to be scientifically and evidentially based. One cannot open a veterinary school based in unproven methods and expect accreditation (i.e., social acceptance). Plainly, society expects veterinary medicine to base what it does, diagnostically and therapeutically, in science.

The fact that some nonalternative or mainstream therapies are not scientifically and evidentially validated does not falsify or negate this claim. It simply means that medicine needs to do better in that area. As previously noted, alternative practitioners who point out that because some mainstream therapies are not scientifically based, therefore they themselves do not need to be scientifically based, are in essence guilty of a classic logical fallacy, known as *tu quoque* ("you, too"). At most, critics may say that science-based medicine sometimes does not live up to its commitment, but they cannot say that its commitment is wrong. And there is certainly much to criticize as non-evidence-based in standard veterinary practice—pinfiring of horses leaps to mind.

What, then, is science- or evidence-based medicine? Are not anecdotal reports of cures evidence? Don't positive results count as evidence? Unfortunately no, at least not to any significant degree. Consider this example: people may pray for a leukemia cure for a member of their family. Behold, the person is cured. Do we count these stories? If we do, we must count the stories of all those who prayed for a cure and there was no cure! Unless someone is keeping track, no one really knows what to make of such stories.

There are myriad forms of observer bias, from the Rosenthal effect,[2] where people have been shown to find what they are told to expect, to wishful thinking. And physicians and veterinarians are not exempt from these human frailties and are as prone to them as anyone else.

It is for these reasons that the notion of objective, randomized, double-blind clinical trials was developed: to get results that are as objective as possible from human observers; to remove bias, self-interest, expectations, and other deforming variables; to put medicine on a firm and repeatable foundation. Such trials are the "gold standard" of proof. Clearly, suspected clinical advances often occur prior to such trials; such suspected advances also provide fruitful ground for additional testing. Still, gold-standard confirmation should always be the goal before a therapeutic modality is put into general use. This is not a way of singling out so-called alternative medicine; it is a rule that should be applied to all therapies that remain untested even in mainstream medicine. This is in fact a major component of what it *means* for medicine to be science and evidence based.

Another component is equally important. In order to be taken seriously (by science-minded professionals, at any rate), a therapeutic modality needs to be logically compatible with empirical verification and, ideally, compatible with scientific knowledge that currently exists. An example of a modality that is excluded by the former component is talking to the souls of animals to learn how to treat them, which, in fact, some people profess to be able to do. This is logically unverifiable. What would count as evidence for such a claim, given that we do not know what a soul is or if there are any? An example of a modality excluded by the latter component is homeopathy, wherein substances are diluted to the point that they cannot be biologically active according to the known laws of biochemistry. It is, of course, always possible that the laws, or our understanding of them, are wrong, but it is not terribly likely at this point, given the weight of the accumulated evidence. Thus, it should not take Herculean experimental efforts to disprove something like homeopathy. On the other hand, positive studies that may appear to support homeopathy can be reasonably viewed with some skepticism.

In sum, if for no other reason than that society expects medicine to be science and evidence based, and charters veterinary medicine accordingly, it is a violation of veterinary medicine's moral obligation to society to do otherwise. This principle holds equally for unproven accepted treatment modalities as for alternative ones. Nor should the principle be seen or used as a cudgel to preferentially assault putative therapies coming from *any* given source, unless those therapies are fundamentally untestable or totally incompatible with what is considered to be certain in modern science. Still, even in the latter case, it is incumbent on veterinary professionals to keep an open mind.

Thus, with regard to veterinary moral obligations to society, it is wrong to promulgate unverified, non-evidence-based therapies. One must also consider the veterinarian's obligation to his or her peers and the profession, and address the issue of unverified therapies in light of those obligations.

VETERINARY PROFESSIONAL OBLIGATIONS

Society expects medical professionals to base their activities on science-based, empirically validated modalities. But perhaps society is in the process of changing its mind, or is inconsistent in its demands. After all, the American Medical Association reports that consumers are spending billions of dollars on alternative modalities, the U.S. National Institutes of Health are beginning to explore alternative medicine, and the Canadian government allotted one-hundred million dollars (Cd) to the study of alternatives. Why shouldn't veterinary practitioners cash in on this trend, given that clients request it?

There is certainly no moral problem in studying, in a scientific way, putative modalities. Accordingly, the NIH and Canada's approach can be commended, assuming that their investigations are held to rigorous standards. Effective remedies may certainly come from nonconventional sources; for example, pharmaceutical companies have for decades used ethnopharmacologists to search for empirical treatments deployed in native cultures. In addition to studying more novel alternatives, it would also be good to see more money allocated to the testing of conventional therapies taken for granted but not empirically verified. Even studying the animals themselves may lead to sources of useful therapies; there is some evidence that animals seek out therapeutic (and even intoxicating!) biological plants. But discovering remedies in unlikely or ancient places and testing them is a far cry from accepting them uncritically.

Unfortunately, given the temporal and economic demands of running a business and making a living, practicing veterinarians are generally not equipped to test modalities of any sort. Accordingly, they usually rely on research institutions to do so. No matter how robust the data backing their interventions, individual practitioners essentially conduct uncontrolled individual experiments and rarely keep data. The best that most practitioners can do is prescribe on the basis of solid scientific evidence that has generally been accumulated elsewhere (which may be more or less convincing) and temper it with their own experience. When it comes to trying new therapies, one can argue that veterinarians should wait until the evidence is in before prescribing unproven modalities.

Still, the question arises again: why not rely on clinical judgment, anecdote, and so on, if no harm is done and if a modality seems plausible? There are several answers. In any untested modality, unrealized harm may be done and what seems plausible may not be. Furthermore, an untested modality may have unsuspected side or long-term effects that may not be immediately recognizable. In some cases, the use of an untested modality may even preclude the use of a tested one.

Still, one of the largest problems with a "what the heck let's try it without evidence" approach is that it opens the floodgates to anyone taking that approach, from faith-healers to voodoo priests to purveyors of snake oil. The only consistently reliable way of demarcating unproven from proven, as has been amply demonstrated, is controlled study. If veterinarians abandon controlled study, why should they enjoy a special position in treating animals? If veterinarians apply a treatment that has not been verified, or embrace treatments to which science is irrelevant, why not have any number of "specialists" treating animals; why not witch doctors; why not chiropractors (who already have demonstrated designs on treating animals); why not anyone who has an anecdote about any sort of modality, including the power of prayer?

It is wrong, vis-à-vis a veterinarian's obligation to the profession, to use or advocate unproven therapies because such use or advocacy implicitly erodes the special status of veterinarians in society. To abandon scientific proof and evidence and replace it with anecdote, attestations, and clinical judgment is to create a situation of medical anarchy and invite a world in which solid empirical verification has no place or pride, and a DVM degree is nothing special. If there are no scientific standards, then there are also no rational grounds for excluding Doctors of Voodoo Medicine from treating animals, or even spiritual healers who treat damaged souls. And this works against the hard battle for scientific credibility and respectability that veterinarians have fought (and largely won) in the twentieth century.

It is important to realize that the concept of medical anarchy is not in and of itself absurd. One could argue that everyone should be allowed to practice whatever he or she wishes without constraint and let the market decide. Such a situation, in fact, prevailed in human medicine during the nineteenth and early twentieth centuries. The problem is that most veterinarians do not realize that this anarchism is the logical outcome of freewheeling use of unproven modalities. Nor would they likely endorse that outcome, since it denigrates veterinary medicine to just one voice in a cacophony of competing hucksters. More to the point, most veterinarians do in fact believe that scientific medicine is in the end superior, and would reject anarchism, not only because it harms veterinary medicine, but also—and primarily—because of the incalculable harm and suffering anarchism would bring the unfortunate animals treated by unproven—and nonfunctional—modalities.

Thus, as regards veterinarians' obligations to their peers and to the profession, the use and advocacy of unproven therapies is largely morally unacceptable, as it plays into the hands of those who would undermine the hard-won authority and credibility of veterinary medicine in society and inexorably leads to a loss of quality control in medicine. It is a virtual certitude that even many clients who demand alternative therapies from a veterinarian would see the power in the medical anarchy argument and would not want to see science-based veterinary medicine in free competition with every conceivable outrageous approach to treating animals.

Thus, one should approach the dispensing of nonproven and non-evidence-based therapies with clear understanding of its implications for the status (and well-being) of the profession, and realize that, if one universalizes using unproven therapies whenever one feels like it, the inevitable outcome is totally unfettered relativism. That is the price for ignoring and debasing the hard-edged criterion separating scientific medicine from unconfirmed speculation.

MEDICAL MORALITY

The next set of morally relevant considerations that must be deployed in assessing the morality of medical practice not based in hard evidence is the effect of such practice on animals, the direct object of the veterinary art. Ultimately, the primary moral obligation of a veterinarian is to the animal. The overwhelming majority of veterinarians would most likely affirm that obligation. While the client legally owns the animal, charters the veterinarian's services, and pays the bills (society not yet seeing fit to guarantee animal health), the veterinarian's duty is to do his or her best to heal the animal, or relieve its suffering; dealing with the client, keeping the client happy, is a necessary evil (to put it harshly). As Plato says, the fundamental function of a shepherd is to protect and improve the sheep under his aegis; his role of wage earner is secondary to that mission. The primacy of the animal is almost a given; hence the shock and revulsion at equine caretakers who hurt the animals for insurance money, for example.

When veterinarians are asked whether they perceive their *ideal* role as being more like a garage mechanic, doing whatever the car owner wishes, or more like a pediatrician, working for the child's well-being regardless, in the end, of what the parents want, the answer overwhelmingly given by pet practitioners is "pediatrician." Even for food animal practitioners working for husbandry agriculturalists such as western ranchers when dealing with sick calves, the answer is frequently the same.

So, viewed in this light, what issues does using unproven therapies on a sick or suffering animal raise? The most obvious issue is: Should one use an unproven therapeutic modality when there is a modality available that is safe and efficacious? The answer is simple—one obviously uses what is known to work! As one veterinary pain specialist put it bluntly: "If a client demands some unproven alternative for pain control, for example, post-surgically, when there is a known effective treatment, for example an opiate analgesic, it is grossly immoral to use something unproven that might not work." He might have added, "No matter what the client wants." After all, the client generally comes to a veterinarian for his or her expertise, not to tell him or her what to do. It is as absurd for the client to dictate therapy as it is for a family member of a sick baby to tell an internist, "Why don't you try Dr. Sleaze's Snake Oil?"

While it is neither necessary nor desirable to antagonize a client, there is nothing wrong with firmly explaining the difference between proven and unproven therapy and what the distinction is based on. In fact, the more clients understand about this difference, the more they comprehend scientific validation. They will be less likely to be persuaded by anecdotes of the form, "So and so said her dog had cancer and mudpacks fixed it." But in any such discussion, the fundamental principle of all medical ethics, "Do no harm," must be made clear. In that vein, following an unsubstantiated rumor about an unproven therapy is generally not in the best interests of the animal.

What if the client says, "What harm will it do to try this anecdotally based therapy?" The answer depends on the circumstances. Most obviously, it must be assured that the treatment does indeed do no harm, or at least the risks of the treatment should be known. Sprinkling holy water into the dog's water-dish is unlikely to do any damage. But stopping antibiotic therapy for an animal with a bacterial infection where the pathogen is susceptible to antibiotics, in favor of holy water, homeopathic remedies, or untested herbs is clearly harmful, and thus wrong.

But what if no one knows the effect and the client is willing to use the alternative modality he or she heard about as an adjunct to what the veterinarian is doing, that is, as something that is complementary to established therapy? What if no evidence-based treatment remains with which to treat the animal?

In such cases, the veterinarian should look into possible dangers of the therapy, and discourage trying it if there is any possible risk and no known benefit. If one is reasonably certain the therapy will do no harm, it is reasonable to continue to work with the client to help monitor the animal's condition and make sure that wishful thinking on the client's part is not selectively ignoring untoward effects, or that the animal's condition is not deteriorating while each new idea is being tried. However, it is also important that veterinarians not provide clients with false hope (see chapter 6).

Veterinarians must not lose oversight of the animals in their care so that they can be vigilant for negative changes. Providing an unproven therapy on request might be rationalized as one way to maintain that vigilance. However, it is possible to maintain vigilance and not profit directly from the application of an unproven therapy, by charging for one's time monitoring the animal instead of charging for the therapy. Whatever decisions an individual makes, it is usually wisest to tell the client the truth, including making the point that the animal may get better after treatment without the treatment having had anything to do with it! Only well-controlled studies can conclusively demonstrate causality.

For the animal's sake, one should not sever a working relationship with a client lightly, no matter what therapeutic demands the client makes. Still, such demands can cause ethical dilemmas for practitioners. In fact, the problem of medical professionals monitoring unproven therapies has arisen for the human pediatric community. These professionals are often faced with situations where clients are (understandably) desperate to try anything after all conventional therapies have failed.

The American Academy of Pediatrics Committee on Children with Disabilities has developed guidelines entitled "Counseling Families Who Choose Complementary and Alternative Medicine for Their Child With Chronic Illness or Disability."[3] These guidelines are reasonable, and conceptually address many often-neglected aspects of disease and treatment. While acknowledging that all medical therapies, conventional or alternative, should be science and evidence based, the guidelines wrestle sympathetically with the mind-set leading desperate people to seek such therapies. They are of great value to veterinarians who embrace the pediatrician model.

The guidelines stress the need for medical professionals not to relinquish their ability to influence treatment and serve the best interests of the child, that is, to retain their Aesculapian authority in their relationship with parents. That does not mean endorsing therapies that might be dangerous, but it does mean not relinquishing one's medical purview over the child. That in turn means being extremely sensitive to parental frustration, desperation, and overwhelming desire to do something. The practitioner should study the alternative modality sought by the client and, in a sympathetic way, critically evaluate the scientific basis of and evidence for the therapy, and forthrightly explain the likelihood of success as he or she sees it. This is likely to entail a discussion of types of evidence, the weakness of anecdote, the compatibility with known laws of nature, and so on. Even more important, the practitioner should communicate possible dangers of these therapies:

> Alternative therapies may be directly harmful by causing direct toxic effects, compromising adequate nutrition, interrupting beneficial medications or therapies, or postponing biomedical therapies of proven effectiveness. Indirect harm may be caused by the financial burden of the alternative therapy, other unanticipated costs (e.g., the time investment required to administer therapy), and feelings of guilt associated with inability to adhere to rigorous treatment demands. If a child receiving alternative therapy is at direct or indirect risk of harm, the pediatrician should advise against the therapy. In some circumstances, it may be necessary for the pediatrician to seek an ethics consultation or to refer to child welfare agencies. If there is no risk of direct or indirect harm, a pediatrician should be neutral.[4]

In order to assure that animals come to no harm, veterinarians must be even more skillful than pediatricians in displaying sensitivity to the client and in deploying their Aesculapian authority, the authority that they possess by virtue of being the treating doctor, as animals do not have the legal protection children do (discussed later).

The pediatric guidelines also suggest that practitioners should discuss improving quality of life for their patients. This can mitigate the hopelessness that leads people to "try anything." Directing the family to support and advocacy groups relevant to the disease in question can be of value in this regard. In addition, the practitioner should not be cavalier in dismissing the alternatives, but empathetic and open, not defensive. If the client insists on adopting an alternative modality, the practitioner should not disengage, but should "offer to assist in monitoring and evaluating the response" in a critical but sympathetic way. In this way, the veterinary clinician can give primacy to the well-being of the animal, yet avoid alienating the client who ultimately captains the animal's fate.

MORAL OBLIGATIONS TO CLIENTS

The next category of moral problems that must be addressed concerning unproven therapies relates to the veterinarian's moral obligations to the client. In the end this is probably the most difficult moral area to deal with, as clients can well stand in the way of effective treatment for animals, regardless of how much they love them. Ultimately, in the eyes of the law, the owners have virtually complete control over their animals, with the exception of the laws barring overt cruelty and outrageous neglect. Owners may choose not to treat sick animals, may choose to euthanize a sick animal, may opt for any bizarre therapy they choose including—and this is a true example—a veterinarian who allegedly talks to animals' souls asking when they wish to be euthanized. This creates, of course, a major problem for veterinarians embracing the pediatrician model mentioned earlier, because the veterinary clinician does not have the power of law behind him or her, the way a pediatrician does. For example, the pediatrician can go to court to force treatment, prevent treatment not in the interest of the child, and, of course, parents cannot elect euthanasia.

So, although veterinarians may see their role as analogous to pediatricians, society (i.e., the legal system) has not yet caught up with the ethic underlying that view, though many if not most members of society would probably agree with it. It is for this reason that veterinary medicine is even more of a people profession than human medicine—one's power to act as an animal advocate depends on the power of persuasion and the ability to deploy one's Aesculapian authority successfully.

Aesculapian authority is the enormous power and authority possessed by medical professionals. Originally discussed in reference to human physicians,[5] its application to veterinarians has also been discussed.[6] In essence, Aesculapian authority is the uniquely powerful authority vested in those that society perceives as healers, historically traceable to the time when medicine was inseparable from magic and religion. It is Aesculapian authority that licenses a medical practitioner to handle a patient with greater intimacy than a sexual partner may. Physicians may probe all parts of the body of patients of either gender, with barely a "by your leave." They tell a patient they must enter an otherwise forbidden area rather than ask for permission. Aesculapian authority confers the sick role, allowing patients escape from responsibilities of work, school, or family. Such authority also compels patients to ingest vile nostrums and medications; surrender spinal fluid to painful procedures; change one's eating or sleeping habits; submit to moral lectures on child rearing; surrender blood, urine, or fecal material; be immobilized; undergo surgery preceded by imposed loss of consciousness; even change one's temperament. What would be dismissed as "torture," in the absence of Aesculapian authority, is meekly accepted by even the most powerful in its presence. As one physician said, "As a physician, I can get almost anyone to do whatever I tell him or her. If a captain of industry or a general or a senator comes to me with an illness, I can order them, as a therapeutic modality, to dangle their naked butt out of a window on the top floor of the Empire State Building, and they will do so." In fact, Aesculapian authority is far and away the most powerful authority in society—even kings, politicians, and dictators submit to medical authority they don't understand and can be scolded and ordered about by physicians.

This authority derives from a combination of traits—sapiential (i.e., special wisdom and knowledge); moral (deriving from the overwhelming moral imperative to heal, relieve suffering, and retard death); and charismatic (derived from the fact that medicine is still related to magic in the eyes of the scientifically and medically naive; i.e., most people). The latter explains why physicians may appear to be threatened by dealing with medical students, veterinary students, or veterinarians—they know too much! Other members of the medical community further reinforce Aesculapian authority, for example, in never calling each other by first names around a patient and almost never directly challenging the pronouncements of peers.

There are, however, strict limits to such authority. For example, it must be deployed to further the best interests of the patient; pursuit of any other end—such as extracting sexual favors from a patient—represent a clear-cut abuse of that authority. This creates ever-present moral problems of abuse of authority for physician/researchers. As one prominent physician researcher said: "Informed consent is a joke. I can extract informed consent for questionable experimental procedures not in their best interest from damn near any patient" [by deploying my authority].

Virtually everything said of physicians increasingly holds true of veterinarians. Indeed many people seek personal medical advice—even assistance—from their veterinarians, who may be held in higher esteem in society than are human medical doctors! These people also confer a sick role on animals and absolve the animals of tasks and responsibilities (particularly with companion animals, but also with working animals like horses), approach animals with great intimacy, perform complex and delicate operations on them, and so on. The primary difference between veterinarians and physicians is that a veterinarian almost always works through a third party, the client and owner, whereas physicians usually work directly with their patients. (The exceptions include pediatricians or those who practice gerontology or psychiatry—they too must often deal with a third party.) But the key point is that, morally speaking, neither pediatrician nor the companion animal veterinarian owes primary allegiance to the third party. Their moral duty is to the patient—they are obliged by the nature of their profession to act in the best interest of the patient. Consequently, they need to avoid orders or requests from the third party that are not in the best interest of the patient.

Aesculapian authority is most likely the veterinarian's most powerful tool for getting clients to act in the best interest of the animal. But there are two ways that this authority can fail. First, a veterinarian can deploy it in favor of unproven therapies, where a proven therapy exists. This is clearly immoral, given what has been said about obligation to the animal and obligation to society to be science based.

The more difficult case occurs when a client is imbued with an ideology refractory to a veterinarian's Aesculapian authority. To take a simple example, consider a suffering cancer animal where there are no realistic options except euthanasia. Despite many veterinarians' opinions that euthanasia decisions should be left up to the client, there are cases where the client refuses to let go, preferring to try myriad unproven therapies. In such a case, a veterinarian's obligation to the animal suggests that a veterinarian should consider doing whatever it takes to end the animal's suffering, and pull out all stops to persuade the owner to euthanize, even exceeding the safe limit to pain control, if in the veterinarian's judgment the animal has no positive quality of life left.

The harder case is when the owner is fundamentally committed to alternative medicine as a worldview that is natural, holistic, new age, based in the wisdom of the East, and so on. For example, when a paper defending evidence-based veterinary medicine appeared,[7] nasty missives from some animal-rights-oriented colleagues, who were good scientists, castigated one of the co-authors for embracing science. "You of all people," wrote one such person, "who have criticized scientific ideology for ignoring ethics and animal pain, should not be embracing a view that requires scientific evidence for therapies, because that leads to more animal suffering in virtue of the need for experimentation." In responding, the author pointed out that evidence can be achieved through clinical trials, and not all evidence requires hurting animals or making them sick. Equally important, using unproven therapies could lead to *enormous* animal suffering if they don't work! In the eighties, "true believers" did surgical wet labs on animals using acupuncture (after sedating and strapping the animal down), convinced that anesthesia was adequate. Yet to more dispassionate observers, it was clear that the animals were feeling pain! And, from a larger perspective, criticizing certain aspects of science does not also entail rejecting the whole package.

Ideologues, often highly intelligent and well educated, are difficult to persuade. It is useful to give them a quick primer on why evidence-based therapy is superior to speculation, and how a strong moral commitment to animals forces the choice for evidence-based medicine. If ideologues insist on pursuing a path leading to harm to the animal, it should be resisted as forcefully as possible.

Equally problematic are situations in which evidence-based medicine has been exhausted, the animal is not suffering, but clients refuse to give up because they have heard or read about some unproven therapy and want to try it. Although a veterinarian may be convinced that the therapy will do no harm, he or she may also be convinced it will do no good.

It is important to keep in mind that there are many types of harm. Useless therapies always do harm, by sapping resources, substituting for validated therapies, keeping up false hope, or any combination thereof. Further, claims that a therapy *may* work, if only as a placebo, while perhaps having some validity in human medicine, are hard to believe about animals (although it has been ingeniously argued that there are conceivable mechanisms by which placebos could sometimes be operative in veterinary medicine).[8] Interestingly enough, a recent paper on placebos in human medicine appearing in the *New England Journal of Medicine* argued that there was little evidence in general that placebos had powerful clinical effects, although there may have been possible small benefits in studies with continuous subjective outcomes and for the treatment of pain (which has a subjective psychological component). The authors concluded that outside the setting of clinical trials, there is no justification for the use of placebos.[9]

In any event, what should a veterinarian do if a client demands essentially harmless, but probably worthless, therapy? Perhaps the best one can do is articulate one's reasons for rejecting the therapy in question, but, as the pediatric guidelines cited above suggest, one should not relinquish the client (and the animal) totally to the alternative therapist. Ethical veterinarians should continue to work with their clients, in part to help assure that unscrupulous practitioners of alternatives do not financially bleed them and in part to keep the client focused on objective milestones that signify efficacy or lack thereof.

THE VETERINARIAN'S PERSONAL OBLIGATIONS

The final ethical category relevant to these discussions is the veterinarian's obligation to himself or herself. Here the issue is straightforward. A practitioner must factor into all such decisions his or her own comfort with a therapy. If he or she is uncomfortable in working with a non-evidence-based practitioner, he or she should not do so, and perhaps should refer the client to another practitioner who will monitor the therapy. On the other hand, if he or she is extremely persuaded of the safety and efficacy of a new but unproven modality, for which one can see a reasonable theoretical basis and has reasonable evidence that it will do no harm, he or she can proceed with it, provided one explains to the client that this attempt is experimental and unproven, obtains informed consent, and most important, does not profit more than breaking even from the attempt. If one does this, however, one should be cognizant of the singular lack of power of such an experiment and should, if one does get encouraging results, do all one can to get the modality tested in a proper experimental setting.

CONCLUSIONS

A variety of ethical vectors militate in favor of veterinarians depending on evidence-based medicine. It is what society has chartered them for; it provides the animal with the best chance of cure or control of pain and suffering; it best meets the client's ultimate desire for the animal to get better; and it secures the profession's status as based in empirical verification. In limited cases, one can deviate from these prima facie moral commitments, but this should not be done cavalierly or for profit.

5

Placebos and Perceptions of Therapeutic Efficacy

Two rationales are commonly employed to justify the use of "alternative" treatments. First, it may be held that even if they don't cause direct treatment effects, they may provoke a "placebo response," with the implication that such a response is somehow beneficial. Second, it may be felt that even if such therapies are ineffective, they may provide hope in a difficult situation, with the implication being that hope, under any circumstances, is good.

On their surface, such rationales are extremely persuasive. After all, one would not want to avoid *any* effective therapy that might help an animal recover, or at least obtain relief, from an otherwise intractable condition. Indeed, it would be clearly unethical for a medical professional to advise against the use of an effective therapy, no matter what its source. Nor would it seem to be prudent to unduly discourage clients, for whom maintaining hope may have important psychological benefits, at least initially, as it may encourage them to stay in touch with their veterinarian and, indirectly, assist in the best ultimate resolution of a clinical situation.

Effects that may be generally, although not necessarily directly, attributed to placebos are ubiquitous. There are undoubtedly shades of placebos in everyday veterinary practice, where complaints can often be vague and treatments may be imprecise. The importance of the perceived value that can come from simply receiving a therapy is shown by the fact that reportedly successful veterinary practices may be based on these values alone, such as with homeopathy, chiropractic (at least for illness), and probably most of acupuncture and herbal therapy, therapies that have provided no established cure for any single condition.

Historically, people consulted doctors even when bleeding and purgation were the basis of mainstream medical practice; remedies and explanations were often much simpler than is the situation today. Whether remedies did anything or not likely mattered little in the context of the minor, self-limiting, or, on the other hand, otherwise untreatable complaints for which they were used. The therapies had credibility in the mind of the patient and they were dignified by widespread usage; this was all that was needed in order for them to be perceived as being effective. Indeed, when any treatment is applied, some of the perceived benefit may be due to placebo-like effects, at least on the owner of the animal, if not on the animal itself.

On the other hand, hope induces feelings of control and optimism that may help clients feel as if they are doing something for their animals. Such optimism may lead to better compliance in the administration of medications, or may lead people to regularly follow prescribed interventions. However, people may expect an unrealistically high payoff from interventions based merely on hope. While hope for improvement may occasionally be warranted, it is important to distinguish between realistic hopes and unrealistic expectations, between confidence and overconfidence. Overconfidence and unrealistic expectations breed false hope, which in turn engenders inflated expectations of success and, eventually, the misery of defeat (see chapter 6).

No matter how laudable, the intention to invoke placebo responses may not be achievable, or even reasonable, nor is the goal of providing hope without its downside. There are some excellent reasons why good intentions may not reflect medical reality and may even range to the edges of ethical medical conduct.

WHAT ARE PLACEBOS?

The term *placebo* originates from the Latin for "I will please." The first usage of the word appeared in the thirteenth century, but it was not until 1785 that the term first appeared in a medical dictionary.[1] Later, placebos were defined as "an epithet given to any medicine adopted to please rather than to benefit the patient."[2]

A precise definition of placebo effects is elusive and temporal. Its existence only requires that any perceived improvement follow a placebo intervention. There is no necessary causal link. In general, placebos are also considered to be medical preparations or treatments that have no specific activity against disease.[3] At one end of the spectrum, some people consider placebo responses as changes in bodily functions that follow the administration of an inert therapy. On the other end, placebo responses may merely be the result of the interaction between doctor, client, and/or patient. As such, it might be seen in any sort of medical encounter.

It is sometimes claimed that placebos invoke nonspecific, and generally said to be beneficial, effects. Thus, they are sometimes administered to control groups in experimental studies in order that specific effects of therapy can be distinguished from simple responses to therapeutic intervention itself. Experimental treatments must be shown to be superior to placebo treatments in order to consider that the experimental treatments have been shown to be effective. In this sense, placebos are not only ethical, they are essential.

However, underlying such a simple experimental concept are complex questions regarding placebos and placebo effects. In practice, the placebo concept is somewhat convoluted and unclear. In the modern definition by Grunbaum, a treatment is a placebo when the effect cannot be explained by the theory that describes its activity.[4] Such effects may be deemed "nonspecific," however, very small changes in meaning of the word *nonspecific* have a potentially huge impact on the methodological aspects of the evaluation of placebos, as well as the moral aspects of prescribing such interventions. In fact, there may not be one dogmatic definition of the term *placebo*.

Regardless, there is considerable question as to whether placebo effects actually affect disease outcomes. That is, while there may be positive responses from patients to the administration of placebo therapies, no one has yet shown that such therapies alter the course of clinical disease. As such, people may feel better after inert therapies are administered; however, the course of their condition is unaltered. In the same vein, people may appreciate the fact that a therapy is applied to an animal, however, that does not also mean that the therapy is of benefit, or that whatever is required to apply such therapies is worth the effort. Whatever the definition, it is apparent that some responses lumped together as "placebo" have other, more persuasive explanations. Lumping mundane explanations for well-understood phenomena into the placebo basket further blurs an already murky concept.

Even if placebo administration could be shown to affect the course of disease, important questions regarding its use and application would have to be answered. For example, even if they were to exist, no one knows the range of placebo effects—positive or negative—and no one knows what causes them. Accordingly, how to best invoke them is, at this point in time, something of a moot point. Furthermore, even if placebo effects could be reliably invoked, would it be ethical to prescribe and/or receive payment for an inert therapy designed to invoke them?

WHAT ARE THE ARGUMENTS FOR THE USE OF PLACEBOS?

One argument for the use of placebos is based on the fact that by attempting to eliminate them, veterinarians effectively reduce their therapeutic options. In a therapeutic setting, a veterinarian who would consider prescribing a placebo might very carefully investigate the owner's complaints about his or her animal, as well as the animal's symptoms, and order appropriate diagnostic tests. If the veterinarian is at least reasonably confident that the animals' health problems do not stem from organic disease, he or she might offer the client a pure placebo to give to the animal in order to allay the client's fears while the animal recovers.

As an example, what is an acceptable evidence-based treatment for fatigue? Various tonics (or in equine racetrack medicine, "jugs"), often containing vitamins, are often prescribed for animals with such vague complaints. Are these simply placebos? Probably. Reassurance, support, and explanation will carry a veterinarian only so far, but some clients insist on something to give their animal, or something to do. Alternative medicine is in part a manifestation of this craving for physical treatments, and veterinarians may fear that by failing to provide something, they will lose a client to another veterinarian or to a non-veterinary animal caretaker. However, as discussed previously, satisfying this craving carries its own ethical considerations.

Another argument that also may be made to justify the employment of unlikely and/or unproven therapies is based on the premise that they may at least invoke a placebo response. These arguments may be generally summarized as, "Even if they don't work, a placebo effect may still be invoked, which may be good." Otherwise stated, the argument for use of the therapies might be rendered as:

> *Premise 1*: Therapies that may not have direct physiological effects (that is, that don't work) may still produce a placebo effect in a patient.
>
> *(Unstated) premise 2*: A placebo effect is better than no real or perceived improvement in a patient's condition.
>
> *Conclusion*: Therapies that may produce placebos are worthy of consideration OR (alternative conclusion) therapies that may produce placebos are valuable.

The problem with the argument, as stated above, is that the premises on which it is based may be false, if for no other reason than that there may be negative effects from prescribing placebos (nocebos), and their occurrence cannot be predicted.

DO PLACEBO EFFECTS AFFECT DISEASE OUTCOMES?

In spite of a large body of work regarding placebos and placebo effects,[5] it is still not generally accepted that placebo effects, in the sense of a physiological response to an otherwise inert stimulus that alters the course of disease, truly exist. The concept of a placebo received popular attention for the first time in 1955. Enthusiastic explorations and expositions of the placebo effect followed for roughly the next 20 years, but by the 1970s, little discussion about such effects was being conducted. Placebo effects were resurrected in the 1980s and have again found a position of prominence in the medical lexicon.

The foundation work for the current interest in placebos was "The Powerful Placebo," published in 1955 by Henry Beecher. Beecher estimated that 35 percent of patients, in 15 trials with different diseases, received satisfactory relief from placebo administration alone. This figure has been widely quoted and the paper is still one of the most frequently cited references in placebo literature. However, it was later shown that this average, even if it is accurate, most likely conceals a wide variation in placebo response among individuals.[6]

However, in 1997, the 1955 article was reanalyzed.[7] In this reanalysis, researchers were unable to find any evidence of a placebo effect in any of the 15 studies cited in the original paper. They did note that there were many confounding factors that could account for the improvement noted by the participants in the various trials, but they concluded that there was most likely no physiological placebo effect at all.

A more recent carefully conducted meta-analysis failed to show that a physiological placebo effect exists. The study reviewed the medical literature from 1946 forward and found 130 studies in which a placebo or dummy-treatment group was compared to a no-treatment group. Of these, 114 were evaluated by means of a formal meta-analysis (a systemized study of studies). The meta-analysis was not able to show that placebo treatments (when compared to no treatment at all) changed objective symptoms of disease.

In the meta-analysis, clusters of studies dealing with the same disease or symptom were evaluated. The studies on pain, a condition for which placebo treatments are commonly employed, did show some placebo effect, but other statistical analyses turned up evidence of bias in these studies. The meta-analysis concluded that either there is no direct physiological placebo effect in treating pain, or the size of the effect was very small. The effects of psychological placebos such as conversations and unstructured doctor-patient relationships were examined, but they did not produce effects that were significantly different from physical or pharmacological placebos. Overall, the study casts significant doubt on whether placebo effects affect disease outcomes.[8]

WHAT ALTERNATIVE EXPLANATIONS EXIST FOR PLACEBO EFFECTS?

There are many ways that false impressions of placebo effects may be produced. It is critical that these factors be accounted for prior to concluding that placebo effects are something that can be reliably, or even occasionally, invoked.

Spontaneous Improvement

Some conditions simply get better on their own—indeed, it has been estimated that at least 70 percent of all acute infectious diseases will improve with no intervention whatsoever.[9] This can even include diseases such as cancer, a phenomenon for which biological mechanisms such as the normal outgrowing of blood supply provide ready explanation for regression or remission, but for which psychological and psychosomatic theories and spiritual ideas may receive credit.[10]

Regression to the Mean

Many chronic conditions have their "ups and downs." If treatment is initiated while the clinical signs are in a down cycle, that treatment has the opportunity to coincide with an improvement that would have occurred anyway. This phenomenon is known as regression to the mean.[11]

It is crucial for anyone engaged in evaluation of medical treatment (conventional or alternative) to understand regression to the mean and take it into account. When a series of quantitative measurements or assessments is being made on an animal over time (pain, flexibility, blood sugar, blood pressure, cholesterol, temperature, growth rate, white blood cell count, etc.) and there is some small fluctuation of the numbers occurring at random (as is true for the above examples), one is not likely to get *precisely* the same numbers from day to day. When an unusually extreme value for that parameter (either high or low) occurs without obvious explanation, the next measurement in the series is more likely than not to be back in the direction of the average, in other words, to "regress toward the mean," simply by random fluctuation. Unfortunately, in human decision making in clinical practice, both patients and doctors are misled into an intervention at the point of those fluctuations.

For example, a client might say, "My dog has had this pain for weeks but it's really bad today so I finally made an appointment to get it checked." Alternatively, a veterinarian might say, "We've been watching your horse's renal function tests over the last two years and it's fluctuated a bit, but this level is a bit higher and I think we should consider fluid therapy to see if we can get those tests down to normal." Regardless of the intervention (in the examples above, fluid therapy or nonsteroidal anti-inflammatory drugs; an herbal remedy or acupuncture), the thing being measured may improve the next time it is measured, confirming that the treatment seemed to work.

The best way to avoid being misled by regression to the mean is use of carefully chosen control groups or intervals and a sufficiently large number of patients or measurements. This is often the most important aspect of research design and can make a study reliable or worthless. On an individual case basis, however, regression to the mean can be confused with a placebo effect.

Hawthorne Effect

The Hawthorne effect is commonly referred to as a change that results simply from participation in an intervention.[12] The term comes from studies initiated in 1924 by the management of the Hawthorne plant of the Western Electric Company in Chicago, Illinois. Workers were told that different lighting levels were being investigated for their effect on production. Production appeared to increase with both increases and decreases in ambient lighting, although the extent of such production increases has been questioned.[13] Investigators concluded that people do better when they think someone is paying attention to them. Things such as positive attention, new ways of interaction with animals, or even the possibility of higher incomes on the part of veterinarians are certainly persuasive explanations for perceived improvements following therapeutic interventions.

Additional Treatment

Alternative medical treatments are often given concurrently with standard treatments (as such, they become complementary or integrative). Curiously, the most unusual therapy often receives credit for the clinical improvement, whether the improvement is real or perceived.

However, administering treatments one on top of the other runs the risk of being unethical if there is no demonstrable advantage to giving (and charging for) the extra treatment. Usually there are certain things that animals need with regard to their care (feed, water, etc.). However, when fees are charged for services beyond those that are clearly needed (such as when an unproven complementary treatment is added to a regimen of proven therapies), a trusting client may rapidly find himself or herself with a bill that is far larger than that which he or she had hoped to pay. Neglecting cost considerations can directly harm clients and indirectly harm patients if finite resources are wasted on ineffective therapies, thereby depriving animals of care from which they might ultimately benefit. This is both inefficient and unethical.[14] At present, even if such additions are satisfying, there is nothing to support the idea that adding unproven CAVM therapies to a proven effective treatment system does anything more than cost the client money.

Conditioning

Conditioning theory proposes that bodily changes result following exposure to a stimulus that previously produced that change. This is perhaps the most intuitively acceptable explanation for any placebo effects in animals. Indeed, animal studies support such a model for placebo effects, starting with the first descriptions of salivating dogs by Pavlov.[15] Both human and animal studies support the idea that conditioning forms some basis for placebo responses.[16] Since conditioning requires learning, it would be expected that repeated visits to a practitioner might increase the strength of the association between learned stimuli and response to treatment. On the other hand, in chronic and/or incurable conditions, long-term negative conditioning from previously unsuccessful conventional treatments may provide a client with much optimism regarding unconventional ones.

Expectancy

Expectancy theory proposes that bodily changes may occur to the extent that the person receiving the therapy expects them to. There is considerable overlap between expectancy and conditioning, because learning is one of the major ways that expectancies are formed. To the extent that therapies are expected to provide relief from disease, or at least provide the client and/or veterinarian with a feeling of control over the disease process, they may alleviate adverse mental states. In that regard, unconventional therapeutic modalities offer a panoply of alternative expectations, often uninhibited by physical or chemical laws. In humans, therapies that help restore patient control may evoke therapeutic effects, but studies that investigate the expectancy model in animals have so far not been performed. Still, if an animal were able to form an association between treatment-related signals (the attention and handling received, the way that the owner behaves toward the animal when it is receiving treatment) and the relief of its distress, expectancies of treatment effects might develop (on the part of both animal and owner).

Opiate Theories

This approach is not a model, but a proposed link between the purported pain-reducing effects of placebos and the internal secretion of opioids.[17] No studies documenting such an effect appear to have been performed in animals. However, the association between placebo interventions and the role of various neuropeptides is far from understood. The situation is made even more confusing in light of the fact that endogenous opioid release is postulated as a mechanism of action for such things as acupuncture and chiropractic. Accordingly, it may be that such interventions and placebo effects are inseparable. Still, it is not surprising that therapies that have no pharmacological basis but that affect mental state can stimulate the secretion of endogenous opioids and other mediators. And the fact remains that known methods of increasing endogenous opioids, for example, exercise, which is inarguably beneficial for health, are generally not the primary method of treating disease, nor are special therapeutic claims made for such methods.

Altered Meaning of Disease

Positive placebo responses may occur when the perception of a problem is altered.[18] Positive changes in the meaning of a problem result when one or more of three things occur:

1. The client feels as if his or her problems have been heard, and receives a satisfactory internally coherent explanation of the animal's problem.
2. The client feels as if his or her problems have been handled with caring and compassion.
3. The client feels as if he or she has a sense of mastery or control over the animal's problems.

As such, alternative therapies, given by a caring and compassionate administrator, have the potential to significantly influence the client's perception of the animal's problem, whether the problem has actually been affected or not. For example, a "traditional Chinese" approach to a problem may allow clients (and veterinarians) to feel as if they are able to approach an incurable complaint from an entirely different direction (from the East, as opposed to the West, as it were). This is satisfying for both the veterinarian, who is able to escape the "limitations" imposed by naturalistic explanations for health and disease, and the client, who is able to do something else to "help" the animal. Even if nothing of benefit is done for the animal, such an interaction is likely to be satisfying for the human participants.[19]

Practitioner Characteristics

Those who practice alternative approaches to medicine are generally less bound by the confines of scientific objectivity than are other practitioners, and their sensibilities are often more optimistic and positive.[20] Positive interactions between people and their doctors tend to produce faster recoveries from conditions that have symptoms but no abnormal physical signs,[21] and there is every reason to believe that such interactions might affect perceptions of veterinary treatment effects, as well. Furthermore, unrestrained by conventional diagnoses and treatments, CAVM practitioners should be more likely to produce diagnoses that match their clients' worldview. When considering that as many as 40 to 60 percent of human patients may never receive a concrete diagnosis[22] (one could argue that the percentage might be even higher in veterinary medicine), alternative diagnoses may help change the circumstances of disease and help people cope, accordingly.

In addition, most CAVM practitioners offer a smorgasbord of treatment schemes. The notions of holism contained in alternative veterinary medicine are extremely broad and indeterminate and, in a sense, treatment schemes targeted at such notions (e.g., considering the animal in its environment) cannot fail.[23] Even if an animal's clinical signs are not directly ameliorated, it is likely that something positive will occur—even if it is only in the client's mind—and the intervention will receive the credit. Alternative practitioners, their diagnoses, prognoses, and treatment scheme(s) may very effectively change the perception of disease and lessen the threat of the unknown and also allow for enough ambiguity to allow for a steady stream of fresh treatment approaches.[24] Whereas practitioners of scientific medicine and its alternatives both have a special status in the practitioner-patient interaction, alternative practitioners have the advantage of always having a ready intervention.

Do Placebo Effects Exist in Animals?

Whether or not placebo effects exist in human medicine, there is little evidence that they exist in animals.[25] In general, placebo responses seem to require that the patient being treated recognize that there is an intentional effort to treat. It is generally felt that animals lack the ability to comprehend such intentions, and they would not be able to participate in such placebo-generating experiences as the power of suggestion or the hope of recovery. Still, such things as conditioning and expectancy, which have been demonstrated in animals, might serve as reasonable explanations for purported placebo effects in animals. Regardless, the hypothesis that a healing or therapeutic effect can be dependably provoked as a result of conditioning cannot be supported at this time.

The Effect of Human Contact

There is research that demonstrates that human contact has measurable effects on animals. Petting by humans reduces heart rates in dogs[26] and horses[27] and causes major vascular changes in dogs.[28] Gentle handling increases productivity in dairy heifers[29] and increases reproductive efficiency in sows.[30] Thus, it is plausible that human-animal contact might play an important role in the observed responses to therapeutic interventions. On the other hand, handling may also be stressful to animals, so responses to handling may not necessarily be beneficial. Regardless, human contact can invoke responses from animals, and animals may behave quite differently when they are not being observed. Thus, it is important to separate handling effects from effects caused by a therapeutic intervention.

Can Therapies Induce Placebo Effects on Owners?

The reported intensity of subjective symptoms such as pain, fatigue, and depressed mood in an animal may vary over time for all sorts of reasons, not all of which have to do with actual changes in symptom severity. Further complicating such analyses are expectations of treatment effects that might exist on the part of both the animal owner and the veterinarian.

Client expectations can be very powerful motivators. Having participated in a therapeutic transaction, clients generally expect to see some results. Optimistic owners may be more likely to diligently pursue treatments. Even failing obvious results, normal reciprocal responses often result in clients reporting improvement, at least initially, even when no improvement has occurred. At the very least, veterinarians can help clients understand what problems are occurring in the animal—such comfort and reassurance may make a problem easier for the client to deal with.

Good veterinary care should include a healthy dose of understanding. However, all three roles—expert, authority figure, and comforter—are subject to abuse when doctors claim effectiveness for a treatment beyond the evidence in the belief that they are doing the patient and client a favor by inducing a placebo effect to the patient's supposed benefit.

IF PLACEBO EFFECTS EXIST, WHAT ARE THE ETHICAL QUESTIONS REGARDING THE USE OF PLACEBOS?

If it could be demonstrated that placebo effects, that is, nonspecific effects that result in improvement in an animal's clinical condition, did not exist, then it would obviously be unethical to prescribe placebos under the aegis of an active treatment. However, even if such effects could be demonstrated and could be shown to result in improvements in animal health, certain ethical questions would remain. While questions regarding the usage of placebos are complex, most of them can be boiled down to some fairly simple issues.

Deception

The dominant argument against prescribing placebos is that it is immoral to deliberately misrepresent a preparation or therapy of no substantial intrinsic utility as something that should better the patient's condition. Should it be demonstrated that the putative treatment were no more than a placebo, this could seriously damage the veterinarian-client bond that is necessary for a good relationship. A breach of trust can ruin any human relationship, but in medical practice, a serious violation of trust, whether the violator is the veterinarian or the client, can be more difficult to remedy than the illness itself.[31]

Regardless, professionals should know better. Veterinarians who routinely prescribe placebos are really no different than astrologers and psychic healers. Indeed, such medical practice is arguably less ethical than the other two fields. Whereas many (perhaps most) astrologers and psychics believe in the alleged supernatural or preternatural influences they cite, scientifically educated veterinarians should know better. Accordingly, those who routinely administer or prescribe inert placebos or medicinals or dietary supplements in hopes of obtaining a placebo effect lack the excuse of naïve belief.

It should also be kept in mind that eliciting a placebo effect does not *require* deception. That is, therapies or prescriptions may be given with the intent of involving owners in their animal's condition. For example, one might suggest that a client run water from a cold hose on a horse's leg, or that the client massage the back of his or her dog with disk pain. Such prescriptions may not actually be effective, but they are unlikely to cause harm, they involve the client, they cost no money, and they may even provide some benefit.

The distinction between using a placebo dishonestly and prescribing placebos to increase owner compliance is subtle but important. Prescribing placebo therapies would involve deception if a client were charged money for them. One would also not typically charge money for the preceding therapeutic suggestions, nor would one couch them in terms such as "thermal hydrotherapy" or "canine myofascial release" in hopes of getting greater client compliance. If a therapy is no more than placebo, charging money for it under the guise of an effective therapy would be unethical and dishonest.

Veterinarian-Client-Patient Interaction

Almost anything can be a placebo. For example, when a client has seen a veterinarian for a cat with an upper respiratory infection, while the cat may or may not recover as a result of the prescribed medication, some of the relief the client experiences results not merely from the pharmacologic action of the drug but also from the emotional support of the veterinarian-client relationship, the veterinarian's authentication and validation of the illness, and the reassurance that the clinical signs of disease do not reflect a more serious underlying condition.

While this interaction is undoubtedly important, it must not be the sole underlying basis for therapeutic interventions. Indeed, any expert can provide reassurance and support. As such, there is no reason that a veterinarian should be able to provide it more "expertly" than any other perceived expert. In placebo-giving contests between trained professionals and sincere lay people, there is no reason to suppose that the trained professional will necessarily be the winner.

Unpredictable Results

The argument that even a positive placebo effect can be anticipated in some percentage of treated patients is not necessarily valid. In fact, no one can predict the effects of placebo treatment. Placebos can also cause adverse side effects (nocebos). So, the possibility exists that placebo therapies may cause harm. The chance of harm is impossible to estimate, as is the chance of success, since the therapies themselves are, by definition, inert. Prescribing an inert therapy with no reasonable anticipation of treatment effect and with unknown risks is simply engaging in a blind experiment conducted without the benefit of informed consent.[32] Such practice would seem clearly unethical and may possibly be harmful.

Encourage Use of Ineffective Treatments

Placebos may encourage people to use ineffective treatments when more effective treatments are available. Obviously, if a treatment is ineffective, promoting it is counterproductive. Presumably no ethical person would wish for someone to waste time, effort, and money on a therapy that did not work. Furthermore, in the case of incurable or self-limiting diseases, such practice is unlikely to cause harm, unless the therapy itself causes direct harm. However, if a placebo were to be substituted for an active therapy, serious harm, even death, could occur. Such instances are beginning to be reported.

Is It Right to Promote Ineffective or Unproven Remedies?

Unproven remedies are of a different sort. These remedies—which are certainly not unique to alternative medicine—might also be thought of as being of questionable efficacy, that is, data are not available to refute or deny whether they work. Under such circumstances, the therapy still *may* work. However, even if a therapy is questionable or might possibly provoke a placebo response, the question arises as to whether it is right to promote unproven therapies, and if not, why not?

In general, there are two broad categories of debates about therapies. These are particularly applicable to therapies characterized as unconventional or alternative. One category is about facts; the other pertains to values. Debates about facts can generally be split into two categories.

It would seem indisputable that any debate about any therapy should proceed from a basis of truth. It is simply not possible to conduct useful debate if the foundational information on which the debate is conducted is not factual. Sadly, much of CAVM immediately diverges from this basic tenet. For example, acupuncture may be promoted as having been used on animals in China for over four thousand years; this statement is simply false. Indeed, given that writing had not developed in China four thousand years ago, even if the statement were true, it couldn't be proven. However, it's also not true—there's no evidence that acupuncture was routinely practiced on animals even fifty years ago, not in China or anywhere else. In the same vein, subluxations, the lesions targeted by many chiropractors (animal and human), have not been shown to exist; homeopathy has never been shown to be effective for any single condition; and there is no such thing as a negative magnetic pole, claims to the contrary notwithstanding. Numerous other examples could be provided. However, the underlying point is that if one cannot begin from a basis of truth, then productive discourse is not possible.

However, once truth has been established, debates about the facts used to establish truth can be further split into two categories. The first factual category concerns arguments about the standards for judging the facts, that is, the way that people know what they know. This is called epistemology. Although some people may claim that there are other ways of knowing, such as faith, observation, or experience, the fact is that science is the currency of medicine and the standard by which therapeutic claims are judged. "Other ways of knowing" are simply not scientific and have been shown to be inferior to it. Thus, if medicine is to be scientific, then one simply cannot uncritically accept other ways of knowing. Alternatively, if medical practitioners uncritically accept other ways of knowing, then those practitioners are simply not being scientific, and, accordingly, they are less likely to ultimately reach the truth about the utility of various medical interventions.

The second factual category concerns arguments about the applications of science itself. It should be a given that science has proven to be the most reliable standard for judging claims of the effectiveness of therapeutic interventions. However, arguments about the application of science certainly exist. They pertain to such things as how reliable and rational its methods are, how the results obtained from the application of those methods are used, if conclusions drawn from individual investigations are valid, if the data obtained from studies are significant, and so on. These debates are productive. They result in continuing investigations, critiques, and responses. Over time, results from such investigations may or may not be reproduced. When these debates are concluded—and it may take years to reach a conclusion—medicine usually finds itself nearer to the truth about a particular subject.

Debates about values frequently are given less attention than are factual debates, but they are no less important. Curiously, and unlike factual debates, most people generally agree about the majority of the standards involved. That is, the moral standards for judging proper and ethical conduct in medical contexts, including the realm of unconventional treatments, generally meet with agreement. For example, one of the foremost principles of medical ethics is that one should not violate the autonomy of another person, that is, one should not impair another person's ability to choose freely. Another principle on which there is general agreement is that people should do things that are likely to result in some benefit and should avoid things that are likely to cause harm.

These principles should seem obvious to anyone. Still, individuals may differ about the moral judgments made in specific circumstances involving these principles. For instance, while people may agree that they should avoid harming animals, they may disagree about whether or not a specific therapy does, in fact, cause harm. Moral judgments about the use of that therapy might conflict accordingly. Indeed, since moral judgments are simply a combination of a principle and a judgment about fact, they can conflict (and they often do) even among people who agree very much on the general principles. With these distinctions in mind, and despite widespread agreement on the moral standards that apply in the use of treatments, including alternative treatments, promotion of unproven and alternative therapies violates moral standards on a grand scale.

In this instance, there is no quarrel with alternative treatments or the mysterious placebo effect, per se. Not everything is known—many discoveries start off as an unusual proposition, as something that cannot be fully explained. Appropriately, these observations lead to scientific investigation; sometimes such investigations prove fruitful, sometimes they do not. That being said, promoting therapies that are generally unsupported by scientific evidence —and the fact is that the vast majority of alternative therapies lack scientific proof—is another matter entirely.

One of the foremost principles of medicine is that one should do what's likely to cause benefit and avoid what's likely to do harm. This principle is almost *always* violated when someone promotes unproven or placebo treatments. This is because the benefits and risks of such therapies have not generally been assessed—indeed, failing some sort of consistent and acute harm, they cannot be assessed on a case-by-case basis. Thus, when evaluating or commenting on such therapies, scientists generally urge caution and oppose such practices, warning that there isn't enough evidence to recommend a particular therapy. Without good data regarding benefits and risks, it is simply impossible to make a rational recommendation about a treatment. Still, promoters of unproven therapies generally disagree with such caution and may ridicule arguments as being too conservative, too limiting, or too restrictive. In the short term, those promoters may benefit from a rush of people interested in dabbling in their novel approaches—in the long term, much time, effort, and money may be wasted. Without good data regarding benefits and risks, it is simply impossible to make a rational recommendation about treatment efficacy. However, it is also a fact that *any* newly proposed therapy is more likely to be unsuccessful than it is to be successful and, as such, it is reasonable to avoid using such therapies until such time as their true worth has been established.

The other moral principle that is often violated in the promotion of unproven or placebo therapy is autonomy. It is immoral to undermine people's ability to make free and rational choices. The autonomy principle is a cornerstone of medical ethics,[33] but it is not always recognized. For example, experiments on unwitting but compliant people, which have been done in the past, are wrong, not only because they may have harmed people, but because they violated people's autonomy. Such experiments were done without informed consent.

Someone's autonomy can be violated with a lie—or simply by providing misinformation. In the same way that it would be possible to restrict people's ability to choose effectively a safe route through traffic if they were blindfolded, it would be possible to restrict their power to choose effectively if they were given false information. Accordingly, a person's power to choose freely and rationally can be dramatically undermined by promoting treatment options that have unknown or no efficacy. So, when a treatment is promoted based on invalid premises, such as putative longevity (for example, acupuncture has *not* been used on animals for thousands of years), as an alternative to harmful medications or as "natural," personal autonomy is violated. The deck has been stacked in favor of the person choosing the therapy. Whether or not a placebo effect is invoked becomes irrelevant.

It doesn't matter if such a violation is intentional; the effect is the same. There is no moral difference between a veterinarian who assures a client that his or her dog is cured of cancer when, in fact, the dog has only a few months to live and someone who sells an herb as a cure for cancer when there is no reason to believe that the herb is effective. Both are wrong, regardless of intentions.

In the movie *The Truman Show*, the protagonist lives in an encapsulated environment. Every choice that Truman makes is free for him, but his choices are actually controlled. The movie is compelling because viewers recognize that Truman's autonomy is being violated on a massive scale and they believe it to be wrong. But what is the difference between Truman's world and a world where countless health claims are urged upon countless veterinary clients each day, with so many of them being false or baseless? In both worlds, the choices are restricted, autonomy is vanishing, and those who cause the vanishing do wrong.

So, promoting unproven therapies is wrong on two counts. It causes harm and it violates autonomy. Such action is immoral, no matter who does it. As painful as it may be, doing the right thing means letting science catch up to the wishes of the therapist and saying, "I don't know, let's find out."

Breakdown of Professional Authority

There is absolutely no reason professionals should be the only ones who can prescribe placebos, and, indeed, they certainly are not the only ones who do so. Placebos may appear to work because of the healing context in which they are applied.[34] Such scenarios involve care, compassion, and skill in bringing about hope and trust. As such, placebo-type effects might conceivably be produced without actually having administered a placebo therapy.

But many visits to physicians' offices are prompted by self-limiting conditions such as the common cold, and treating self-limited conditions is largely an exercise in futility. One's cold will disappear within seven days if one takes a medicine for it, and within one week if one doesn't. Vague equine performance problems, canine behavioral concerns, or unreasonable preoccupation with ideal nutrition are arguably best treated by a psychologic rather than pharmacologic means.

Placebo-based treatments abound in practitioner caring and thus seduce clients and veterinarians. The satisfaction factor is powerful. Client dissatisfaction due to the veterinarian's unwillingness to prescribe *something* might prompt a switch to a different veterinarian. On the other hand, the ability to provide as many options as possible can keep the client coming back for more.

It is not necessary to provide just *something* to maintain veterinary authority. For example, in seeing a horse with a simple upper respiratory virus, instead of providing antibiotics, veterinarians might instead briefly discuss with the patient the differences between bacterial and viral infections, discuss why using antibiotics inappropriately is hazardous, and give the patient an educational handout that covers how colds are self-limiting and how rest and other comfort measures can make a cold more tolerable. (It would be appropriate to then charge for the time spent.) Similarly, a sedentary dog with arthritis may benefit merely from reduction in weight, increased attention being paid to it, and an increase in exercise level. Adjunctive acupuncture, while pleasing to the client, certainly does not alter the course of disease, may not be helpful in symptom management, and may ultimately be harmful to professional credibility if it turns out that such interventions are no more than placebo. Unfortunately, renegades who espouse such concerns risk losing their patients—and their patients' families, friends, and coworkers—to practitioners who have no qualms about prescribing placebos and who thus may appear more caring.

While one might have hoped that progress in medical research and technology would have obviated the routine prescribing of placebos, bringing a veterinary visit to a satisfactory conclusion might imply that *something* must be done. But what should constitute a satisfactory conclusion to a medical visit? Must a therapy be provided? Client demands are often not made with any medical knowledge whatsoever. For example, when clients see that an animal is sick, they may think that antibiotics are indicated. If that infection is viral in origin, antibiotics are not indicated. While the client may be satisfied because he or she has something to administer to the animal, the practice of prescribing antibiotics as antiviral placebos has the potential for harm. For one thing, this practice may be contributing to the emergence of resistant bacterial infections. Thus, in this case, a veterinarian's refusal to provide an antibiotic to an animal with a viral infection under the guise of giving something because the client has requested such sets up a dilemma between the right thing to do and the desire to satisfy the client. Giving in to client demands in this case is potentially harmful, socially unacceptable, and wrong.

Finally, if the therapeutic use of placebos were legitimized, the public would become aware of the event in short order and be outraged by it. The take-home message for patients would be that physicians' trustworthiness is relative. Patients would, in effect, hear from their veterinarians: "Yes, I know I gave you a placebo last week, but now I am (really) telling you the truth." Without trust, the doctor-patient relationship would be in free fall.

A Pill for Every Ill

Placebo therapy reinforces the erroneous and harmful notion that there is a pill for every complaint. Use of placebo-based therapies encourages the unhealthy belief that all symptoms have pharmacologic antidotes or need some sort of medical intervention. Placebos should not be used as substitutes for conversations between veterinarians and clients, even when such conversing would be difficult.

Prescribing placebos can also be a convenient "exit strategy" for doctors treating persons with chronic or intractable symptoms, giving the patient something to do while doing nothing to directly address the animal's condition. However, this sort of rationalization, no matter how well intentioned, is also dishonest. Good intentions are no excuse for using placebos therapeutically. Indeed, it is not possible for a client to give informed consent to nonexperimental placebo administration. Snake oils and their pseudoscientific relatives should be anathema to veterinarians.

The Requirement to Provide Effective Therapies

It would seem that the purpose of veterinary medicine is to do more than merely administer treatments in the hopes of invoking ill-defined, inconsistent, and perhaps even nonexistent responses. In the absence of direct evidence from placebo-controlled, double-blind trials, it is reasonable to regard any new or unusual form of treatment as potentially a form of psychotherapy. This is the reason the debate over the need for proper scientific trials has become a central debate in the world of alternative medicine.

The implications of finding that any particular CAVM therapy relies largely on the placebo effect and has little or no treatment-specific effect must be seriously considered. If CAVM is claiming that it has a specific value for a particular condition, then it must be shown that there is a treatment-specific effect over and above the placebo effect. People are entitled to know how they are spending their money. It is also important from the veterinary profession's point of view, as various practitioners consider spending their money to become "certified" in various CAVM therapies.

If placebo effects could positively improve objective biological measures of health, then treatments that enhanced such effects could be considered worth attaining in their own right. However, there is probably little justification for supporting the wider advocacy of any technique that relies solely on the placebo effect since it depends so critically on the particular beliefs of that particular person at that particular time.

CONCLUSIONS

Invoking placebo effects cannot be generally used as a justification for employing therapies of no proven benefit. Indeed, most evidence suggests that, in general, placebo infections do not have cliniclly important effects.* Whether such effects occur or not, therapies must be more than placebos. Conversely, placebo responses may be invoked with any therapy—it is not necessary to pretend that effective medications are being provided to incorporate them. Professional credibility is ultimately at stake.

ACKNOWLEDGMENT

The authors would like to thank Asbjørn Hrobjartsson, PhD, for his kind assistance in reviewing this chapter.

---

*"Although placebo interventions are often believed to improve patient reported and observer reported outcomes, this belief is not based on evidence from randomised trials comparing placebo treatment with no treatment. A 2003 analysis of 130 randomised clinical trials investigating 40 clinical conditions which had a no-treatment control group was conducted to assess the effect of placebo interventions. There was no statistically significant effect of placebo interventions in eight out of nine clinical conditions investigated in three trials or more (nausea, relapse in prevention of smoking and depression, overweight, asthma, hypertension, insomnia and anxiety). There was a modest apparent analgesic effect of placebo interventions, but this apparent effect could not be clearly distinguished from bias. "Hrobjartsson, A., Gotzsche, P.C. Placebo treatment versus no treatment. Cochrane Database Syst Rev 2003; (1): CD003974.

6

Hope

A common argument used to support the practice of administering unproven, alternative, or dubious therapies is that it may provide a chance, or at least some hope. In this context, hope is said to be a good thing; therefore it should be encouraged. Hope is a desire, in this case, the desire for improvement in animal health accompanied by expectation of or belief in the fulfillment of that desire.

Providing a therapeutic option is a powerful way to provide hope. Indeed, for human patients, it may even help with resolution of patient complaints. For example, it has been demonstrated that when human patients are affected with symptoms of disease but without underlying organic pathology, they recover at a much higher rate (64 percent to 39 percent) when a diagnosis is provided and assurance that the condition will improve in a few days is given, as compared to when the physician admits to not knowing what the condition is or how long it might last.[1]

Why is hope an important consideration in veterinary medicine? Mostly because people anticipate that by providing some sort of therapy, benefits will accrue to their animal. In the face of a disease, in addition to trying to achieve a cure, people may try to provide therapy because it will make the animal less painful, more content, healthier, or more likely to recover more quickly from the disease process itself. In general, even if a therapy is inert, administering it brings hope to the client. For the veterinarian, providing options may bring admiration or appreciation from the client and provide internal advantages such as pride and self-confidence. The combination of medical ignorance on the part of the consumer and uncritical enthusiasm on the part of the practitioner allows practitioners of alternative medicine to promise wonders—or at least help—in situations where more circumspect veterinarians can offer only limited hope. Thus, the major attraction of providing therapeutic alternatives is the anticipated outcome. Moreover, altering something about a therapeutic approach may also be a way of attempting to gain control over animal health.

Alternative interventions are generally applied with goals that can usually be attained. Thus, while the various CAVM modalities may not be promoted as ways to cure disease, they may offer numerous alleged benefits, such as improving animal demeanor, comfort, disposition, or quality of life (to name a few). A disease process may be immutable and resistant to a cure, but symptoms are malleable, and something that may be changed, allowing for at least the *possibility* of therapeutic success. Some changes are relatively easy (e.g., changing diet), whereas others are more difficult (e.g., improving a limp due to osteoarthritis). Presumably, one is more likely to embark upon a change that is believed to be not only possible but also easy to effect; the changes espoused by CAVM therapies often fit such a bill.

However, apparently lost in discussions about hope is the question of to whom the hope is being provided. Clearly, an animal cannot consciously expect to benefit from *any* treatment that is being provided for it. Thus, it is clear that any hope that is being provided is merely for the benefit of the client and/or the veterinarian and not the patient. While interventions may be provided in hope of providing a cure, the condition of the animal must not be ignored while "hopeful" remedies are being applied. Indeed, one of the foremost charges of a veterinarian is to relieve animal suffering—providing nothing but hope in the face of continuing and deteriorating disease states runs the risk of prolonging animal suffering, although perhaps satisfying client and veterinarian. This is clearly unethical.

WHAT ARE THE MOTIVATIONS FOR THE USE OF CAVM?

While no specific surveys appear to have been done investigating the reasons among animal owners for the use of CAVM therapies, numerous surveys in human medicine have identified some of the underlying motivations for the use of alternative therapies in people. These include:

1. Response to alluring claims. For example, suggestions that alternative remedies may enhance immune function or prolong life or cure disease are attractive, even if unsupported, claims.[2]
2. Psychosocial distress in response to troubling medical conditions for which there are no cures.[3,4,5]
3. A desire for a sense of control of disease conditions, which CAVM offers by minimizing sentiments of passivity (that is, people feel as if they are doing something).[6]

4. Fear of death and disease. For example, in human oncology patients, loneliness, pain, and feelings of emptiness enhance such fears; alternative approaches may help in attenuating them.[7]

Thus, the use of alternative modalities in people (and, presumably, CAVM modalities in animal owners) appears to be largely unrelated to issues of therapeutic efficacy. Rather, such use appears to be driven by unmet desires and clients' needs to have their fears heard and understood. To the extent that CAVM practitioners are able to satisfy those needs and desires, one would expect that clients would warmly embrace their practices, even in the absence of evidence of efficacy, particularly when those services are delivered for the treatment of self-limiting or chronic and/or incurable disease conditions. As such, CAVM practices may provide a client with hope—warranted or not—that his or her animal's condition will improve, or at least with reassurance that the client is doing all that he or she can in an effort to treat or prevent disease.

HOPE AND HEALING

Any practice that calls itself medicine, whether it calls itself scientific, integrative, alternative, or complementary, should be aimed at restoring health and alleviating suffering by preventing or treating illness. In such a context, the word *healing* is particularly interesting. While injured and diseased animals may certainly heal in certain circumstances, in the sense of returning to normal, part of CAVM appears to have lost contact with the word *healing* itself. Instead of being concerned with the treatment of disease and injury, CAVM therapies have adopted a broader context for the word. As such, healing holds to the notion that the goals of medicine have to do with making the patient "whole" (the word patient comes from the Latin word *patientem*, "to suffer"). Viewed in this context, many such therapies leave the world of medicine.

Of course, there are many ways to fulfill human emotional needs that lie outside the range of medicine. In addition to physical and psychological well-being, people seek things like health and happiness, spiritual fulfillment, and a balance between labor and leisure. They seek them in many ways: listening to music, praying, working, caring for an animal, reading, meditating, hiking, and being with friends and loved ones. These are all ways that people seek the good life without claiming that they are part of medicine. Nor does anyone feel obligated to prove the value of the various approaches. These are alternatives *to* medicine.

Why is this distinction important? It is important because many proponents of CAVM therapies do not claim that their therapies are alternatives *to* medicine, that they help alleviate client distress, rather, they claim that they *are* medicine. They claim that they not only provide such things as balance and wellness, but that they also treat and/or cure specific diseases. What can be said regarding these claims? If such statements were placed in peer-reviewed medical journals, they would have been challenged along evidentiary lines. However, when they are challenged, CAVM proponents often cry foul.

Problems arise when feel-good notions about balance, holism, and nature begin to encroach on the practice of medicine. Although such concepts may be soothing to some, in general they are virtually devoid of real medical meaning. Indeed, they often conflict with medical reality. Instead of being in accord with generally accepted and well-understood terminology, such notions are generally defined by the person doing the defining. So, for example, a product or service might be said to "support" an organ, to "detoxify the system," or to address any one of innumerable ill-defined or nonexistent conditions. From a medical perspective, such concepts are inherently meaningless.

While these approaches may comfort, provide hope, or even be persuasive to those with a limited understanding of the complexities of medicine, they are ultimately counterproductive. They cheapen the practice of medicine, reducing it to a series of meaningless aphoristic diagnoses with simplistic solutions. Providing hope for medical cures by appealing to vague and immeasurable notions of healing is making an empty promise, even though such notions may be emotionally fulfilling and raise client hopes. If those hopes are unfulfilled, real emotional damage to the client may result. Meanwhile, animals may be forced to endure a series of needless services.

Medicine is not simply talking about living the good life and restoring harmony and balance. Nor can veterinary medicine fulfill every need (human or animal). Yet with respect to whatever veterinary medicine does take responsibility for, it owes a scrupulous attention to empirical data to avoid misinforming and harming patients.

HOPE AND CONTROL

Individuals prefer to feel in control of the well-being of their animals, and providing care for them promotes such feelings. Even when they engage in activities where outcomes are determined purely by chance activities, people who take an active role develop an exaggerated sense of control. For example, those who pick their own lottery tickets instead of having the experimenter assign one to them feel more in control and more confident of a favorable outcome. Similarly, subjects gain a sense of control over an outcome if they are allowed to perform a behavior connected with a chance event, such as choosing a marble out of a hat rather than being given one randomly by an experimenter.[8]

Human cancer patients who perceive that they have more control over their disease are less depressed, even after the effects of such variables as physical functioning and marital satisfaction have been eliminated.[9] Even simply phoning to schedule an appointment with a psychotherapist produces measurable improvement in distressed individuals.[10] There's no reason to believe that such effects would not occur in a veterinarian-client relationship. Incorporating dietary changes, massage, or any other number of putative therapies—be they of real benefit to the animal or not—allows both veterinarian and client to feel more in control of an animal's health. As such, any intervention, be it from a veterinarian, a concerned friend, or an unlicensed animal healer, has the possibility of increasing feelings of control.

REALISTIC VERSUS UNREALISTIC EXPECTATIONS

In order to consider whether or not expectations of therapeutic efficacy are realistic, it's necessary to examine whether the expected outcomes are actually connected to the therapeutic intervention that is undertaken. For some interventions, the predicted benefit may simply result from some alteration in an animal's care. For example, in overweight dogs with hind limb lameness secondary to osteoarthritis of the hip, weight reduction alone may result in a substantial improvement in clinical lameness.[11] Such simple suggestions provide some basis for hope and are reasonably attainable. Still, no matter what is done for the dog, it is not currently possible to restore the arthritic joints to normal—accordingly, a goal to reverse arthritis will ultimately result in failure. When a plausible outcome is desired but cannot actually be achieved, failure is inevitable because expectations are overinflated.

On the other hand, expectations that animals may benefit from manipulation of their energy fields are unrealistic, as such fields have never been demonstrated. Nevertheless, belief in such fields allows for interventions that address them; improvement may thus be as subjective as are the imaginary fields themselves. Certainly, if an animal appears to improve after such interventions, they will almost certainly get credit for the perceived improvement and such therapies may thus be perpetuated.

IS THE BENEFIT OF CONTROL WORTH THE COST?

The advantages gained by feeling in control over an animal's disease process may be considerable, even if the treatment has no effect. As such, the argument may be otherwise stated as, "What is the harm, if the treatment itself is harmless? Why shouldn't people be given a chance to try it on their animals?"

As the argument is framed, even if there were no strong evidence that a treatment is effective, if it were effective, the benefits to animals with otherwise untreatable or uncontrollable conditions would be substantial. Since the costs, in terms of actual physical harm to the animals, are generally low (most CAVM therapies are generally promoted as being safer than mainstream therapies and are likely to be so), on balance, the argument is made that it's best to urge people to try the therapy. The possible benefits are said to outweigh the possible costs. Promoters of unproven therapies may believe that this argument is particularly strong if there is some preliminary evidence for the effectiveness of the therapy, or if the monetary outlay for the treatment is low.

To consider this argument, it must be agreed that a benefit-cost ratio is a good way to judge the issue. Obviously, in any such equation, one hopes that the balance comes out in favor of benefits. But the larger question is, "Is this argument good?"

Unfortunately, it is not. The argument itself is not valid because it fails to consider all the variables in the equation. There are other variables to consider in addition to the fact that a putative treatment may have some enormous possible benefit. Most important, there is the question of probability.

In fact, it would seem unreasonable to judge a treatment based only on weighing its proposed benefit against the potential harm. Such an equation fails to consider the probability that the proposed effects would actually happen. For example, someone might claim that waving his or her hands over a dog lying in a certain direction might cure its prostate cancer. The alleged benefit of such a therapy is enormous. Unfortunately, the likelihood of receiving the benefit is infinitesimally small. If someone were to engage in therapeutic cancer-curing hand waving on a precisely placed canine, and the price for such a service was only ten dollars, would it be worth it? No.

The reason the therapy would not be worth the cost is not because the promise isn't big enough. The promise, curing prostate cancer in a dog, is huge. However, even though the proposed benefit is tremendous, it's not at all likely to occur. However, the cost is a sure thing. If someone wants to have hands waved over his or her dog, there is a price that will have to be paid. On balance, the likely cost, though small, outweighs the unlikely benefit, though great. The fact that the cost goes to the person providing the hand waving—the person who most likely recommended the intervention—also sets up an obvious conflict of interest.

What's the likelihood that *any* given treatment is going to work? The evidence relating to any unproven remedy can't determine that—by definition the evidence is too weak to help us with the probabilities. However, it is possible to make reasonable assumptions. The chances of any new hypotheses being correct are very low, simply because it's much easier to be wrong than it is to be right. The equation $2 + 2 = x$ has only one right answer ($x = 4$) but an infinite number of wrong ones (and that, considering only the integers). For the same reason, the likelihood of new health claims turning out to be true is also very low. Historically, most health hypotheses, when adequately tested, have also been found to be false.

Another, often forgotten issue is one of biological plausibility. When bio-chemical tissue and animal data point to a mechanism of action or demon-strate the desired biological effect, they thereby confer biological plausibility. Unfortunately, many CAVM therapies, such as homeopathy, magnetic thera-py, or Bach's Flower remedies, completely lack biological plausibility. Indeed, for a therapeutic approach to be considered CAVM, it must, almost by defini-tion, be scientifically implausible. A biologically plausible mechanism of action greatly aids in selecting an appropriate dosing regimen and patient population and encourages persistence in the face of disappointing results. But, the stranger and more biologically implausible a therapy, the higher the bar for crediting evidence supporting its clinical plausibility should be set.

Accordingly, many people simply misjudge the probabilities involved in assessing the potential benefits of therapeutic interventions. They either over-estimate the probability of a therapy being effective, they don't consider whether or not it's plausible, or they don't consider such factors at all. They seem to consider that the odds of a particular therapy being effective are close to 50:50, especially if there is some preliminary evidence in its favor. This is simply false. When realistic probabilities and plausibility are plugged into the moral equation about costs and benefits, the wisdom of promoting unproven treatments becomes suspect. Even if an unproven treatment has considerable *possible* benefits, is harmless, and costs very little, it may not be a bargain. In general, given the realistic probabilities, the most likely prospect is that the treatment will be *ineffective*. In fact, the odds are excellent that people who buy the treatment will waste their time and money. The guaranteed costs outweigh the unlikely benefits. Promoting the treatment is not likely to result in a net benefit, but a net harm. The possible benefit of waving hands over the dog with prostate cancer may be great, but the low probability that it will work makes buying it a bad deal. Promoting it would therefore be wrong.

But there's more to the cost than just the probabilities. Although the mone-tary cost can vary tremendously and may not be low at all, it is possible that an individual could apply our equation to himself or herself and rightly conclude that he or she should try an unproven remedy. For example, if *any* possible benefit is worth any possible cost, no matter how implausible the therapy, an individual may choose to employ it. Promoters, however, aren't privy to this information. They can only weigh the probable impact of their actions on other people—not to mention the animals. Thus, in general, promoting unproven treatments does more harm than good.

HOPE AND DIRECT HARM

In considering hope, one must also consider the potential for direct harm (nearly all treatments have potential to cause harm). Unfortunately, for CAVM therapies, the risks and benefits for treatments are generally not well known. Nonetheless, direct harm from alternative interventions has been reported, particularly in human medicine, particularly with the increase in consumption of unregulated medicinal herbs.

INDIRECT COSTS OF HOPE

There is also an indirect cost of hope. That is, while hopefully searching, some people may stop, postpone, or refuse proven therapy, a gamble that may have tragic consequences.

However, in considering hope, one must keep in mind the setting in which hope is given. The animal owner presents an animal with a newly diagnosed condition, which may or may not have a solution. That person is confronted with an expert on whose counsel his or her animal's future depends. On the other hand, the veterinarian/expert sees a patient with a prognosis that may range from completely curable to dismal, with potential benefits of treatment ranging from marginal to quite dramatic. The client counts on the veterinarian to save his or her animal—the veterinarian doesn't want to let the client down. Given this dynamic, it is easy to understand why clients would be willing to try almost anything, and trust in the expert providing the therapeutic options. Still, if it is perceived that veterinarians are merely offering hope, instead of options that have a reasonable chance of success, professional credibility may suffer.

FALSE HOPE

Then there is the problem of false hope. False hope is the dashed promise of hope. False hope can bring very real emotional pain. For reasons previously discussed, false hope is actually more likely than fulfilled hopes. When the costs of false hope are factored in, the argument for promoting unproven therapies becomes even weaker.

Therapies must be provided with realistic predictions for success and based on factual information. Failing such criteria, unreasonable expectations for therapy may be held, both by the client and the veterinarians. If treatment fails, individuals may feel frustrated and despondent, and give up. Unrealistic beliefs that prompt people to try unproven therapies, and unattainable criteria for success, may create a false hope and then dash it. This phenomenon of beginning with high hopes and expectations of successful outcomes is illustrative of a phenomenon that has been termed the "false hope syndrome."[12]

Increased perceptions of control that occur as a result of engaging in new therapeutic directions may lead both veterinarians and clients to feel a false sense of confidence in their likelihood of achieving therapeutic success and to overlook other reasons why success might occur.[13] This, in turn, may engender distorted beliefs about the effects that such treatment may have on other aspects of their lives. When these expectations are not met, the outcome may be disappointment and discouragement.

False hope is, in many respects, a problem of overconfidence. One cause of overconfidence or unrealistic expectations may be inflated promises provided by CAVM practitioners. Groups, books, internet chat rooms, websites, and other sources of information often play into people's fantasies that the answer to their animal's health problem is just around the corner or steeped in some ancient or overlooked traditions. Successful therapeutic outcomes may be routinely promised, despite the fact that there is little evidence for such alleged successes.

Another source of overconfidence is the individual. When people make decisions that involve committing themselves to a particular goal or therapeutic program, "their positive illusions or overconfidence should create a tendency to set goals too high for themselves, with the result that their likelihood of eventual failure increases."[14] Furthermore, failure of a particular intervention may result in what has been termed *cognitive dissonance*.[15] According to this theory, when new information contradicts existing attitudes, feelings, or knowledge, mental distress is produced. So, for example, if a new therapy is undertaken, people are hopeful of seeing an effect. If no effect is seen, mental discord may result. This mental discord may be alleviated by reinterpreting, that is, distorting, the offending input. To have received no relief after committing time, money, and "face" to an alternate course of treatment (and most likely to the cosmology of which it is a part) would be likely to create this kind of internal dissonance. Because it would be too disconcerting, psychologically, to admit to one's self or to others that it had all been a waste, there would be strong psychological pressure to find some redeeming value in the treatment.

Other cognitive distortions contribute to unrealistic expectations. Those who attempt to change certain behaviors have often made similar efforts in the past and are more likely to remember previous successes than failures. Unfortunately, however, the optimism and positive effect that accompanies the initial application of a new therapy may fade away when the realities of incurable or uncontrollable conditions set in.

What happens when hopes are dashed? Generally, feelings of guilt and hopelessness develop. But soon the next therapy appears, bringing renewed hope that this time the condition will finally improve. The ever-expanding smorgasbord of CAVM therapies attests to the sad fact that desire for cures outstrips the ability of medicine to provide them. Still, the pursuit of endless options may start a downward spiral of chasing new therapies, leading only to a waste of money and ultimately perhaps depriving clients of the ability to bring their association with their valued animal(s) to a peaceful and satisfying conclusion.

CONCLUSIONS

Veterinarians do not have the right to define hope for their clients. Their task is to be up front with them, to provide continual comfort and care and allow them to define their own hope. Even the most empathic veterinarians cannot always anticipate the reactions of their clients. Confidence and hope are particularly powerful when outcomes are achievable; hope, the belief that a condition can be cured or controlled, is a powerful factor. However, when the alteration is too difficult or one's expectations are not realistic, confidence may become overconfidence, leading from hope to false hope. In order to replace false hopes with real hope, it is essential to learn to determine accurately the real efficacy of treatments, to establish realistic goals, to keep expectations reasonable, and to develop coping skills to help contend with the setbacks that are normal with efforts to influence biological processes.

7

Scientific Aspects of CAVM

GENERAL CONSIDERATIONS

The first and most basic rule of medicine is "above all, do no harm." This principle has been followed as a major rule of medical ethics since at least the time of the Greek physician Hippocrates (ca. 460–377 B.C.). This precept implies that in treating a health problem, no procedure, device, or therapy should expose an animal to more risk than the risk that the problem itself would pose if it were left untreated.

However, treatment of animals is more than merely a matter of causing no harm. A veterinarian also has a moral and ethical obligation to provide therapies to animals for which there is good evidence of effectiveness. Indeed, society desires and expects that effective therapies are being provided;[1] it's more than just a matter of serving up something that a client wants. Since, for any therapy, establishing proof of efficacy, as well as potential risks and benefits, is an ethical requirement, the salient question becomes, "What is the best way to determine therapeutic safety and effectiveness?"

Veterinary medicine is based on veterinary science. Indeed, the Veterinary Oath avers that the taker will "use my *scientific* knowledge and skills" [emphasis added].* By applying veterinary science, veterinarians should attempt to

---

*Veterinarian's Oath: "Being admitted to the profession of veterinary medicine, I solemnly swear to use my scientific knowledge and skills for the benefit of society through the protection of animal health, the relief of animal suffering, the conservation of livestock resources, the promotion of public health, and the advancement of medical knowledge. I will practice my profession conscientiously, with dignity, and in keeping with the principles of veterinary medical ethics. I accept as a lifelong obligation the continual improvement of my professional knowledge and competence."

ensure that an animal's condition has been accurately and objectively diagnosed, that the treatment being provided is specific for the animal's condition, and that the effects of the treatment are an improvement over merely allowing the disease to follow its natural course. Veterinary medicine is a trusted and respected field in part because of this dedication to objective diagnosis and substantiation of therapies.

Such respect has been hard to come by. In fact, for most of the twentieth century, veterinary medicine struggled to attain scientific status on par with human medicine. The term *horse doctor* was once one of opprobrium. Because medical professionals have laid claim to having great knowledge about medicine based on medical science, society now expects such an approach from medical professionals, and it has been willing to largely give up its right to a free market for health care (in human and veterinary medicine).

Such a societal expectation has been long in coming. Indeed, nineteenth-century Americans were unwilling to yield their private judgment on health matters to physicians—anyone could attempt to heal the sick. It was not until medical professionals established persuasive claims to having special knowledge that licensing laws—abolished in the middle part of the nineteenth century—began to be re-established.[2] The most convincing explanation for this attitude change is the rise of science and technology, with the concomitant increase in the competence of medical professionals.[3] Further evidence of society's expectations is demonstrated by the United States Supreme Court, which has repeatedly upheld and refined the law in regard to the reliability of scientific standards as a benchmark for evaluating legally admissible and credible evidence.[4]

If science is indeed the standard by which effective veterinary medicine is to be gauged, if it is the thing that separates veterinarians from nonveterinarians, then it should also be important to appraise CAVM therapies by that standard. While, in general, veterinary science may trail human medical science in critically investigating the safety and efficacy of various supposed treatments, nevertheless, a substantial body of scientifically sound evidence supporting commonly used veterinary treatments does exist. In cases where direct scientific proof is lacking, such therapies are still based on sound biomedical principles (that is, they are biologically plausible).[5] However, in alternative veterinary medicine, good evidence of effectiveness is almost entirely nonexistent. Indeed, virtually all CAVM therapies are scientifically unproven therapies, almost by definition.[6] In fact, some, such as homeopathy, violate well-established scientific principles, and, as such, can be reasonably regarded as having already been disproved. Therefore, it's more likely on an *a priori* basis that alternative therapeutics will be based on opinion and personal belief rather than on scientific evidence. Of course, if CAVM therapies were proven, they would not be alternative. Rather, they would be among those largely safe and generally effective therapeutic interventions validated by means of rigorous science.

Does basing practice on scientific evidence matter? There certainly are those who would suggest that it does not. Some people may assert that a scientific philosophy of practice has tremendous limitations when it comes to taking care of individual patients. Others have suggested that science and objectivity are themselves merely arbitrary social constructs, and, as a result, anecdote, testimony, and clinical (personal) experience should be given equal weight to scientific lines of evidence, which only *claim* to be more objective. Still others may note that the data gleaned from science may not apply to many of the treatments that are offered to patients in clinical practice, in subgroups of disease, or for various prophylactic interventions, diagnostic decisions, or even psychosocial factors.[7]

Whatever the merits of such criticisms, the relevant question is, "Does providing scientific, evidence-based care improve outcomes for patients?" Unfortunately, there have not been studies that have looked at this question directly, most likely because no investigative team or funding agency has yet figured how to overcome problems such as necessary sample size, blinding, and long-term follow-up that such trials would entail. Furthermore, such a trial would pose serious ethical questions; specifically, "Would it be ethical to withhold evidence-based treatments from a control arm?" That said, outcomes research has documented that patients who receive scientific evidence-based therapies often have better outcomes than those who don't. So, for example, in human medicine, survivors of myocardial infarctions who are given aspirin[8] or beta-blockers[9] have lower rates of mortality than those to whom such drugs are not prescribed. When clinicians use more warfarin, and refer patients to stroke care units, stroke mortality declines by greater than 20 percent.[10] For a negative example, patients who undergo surgery of the carotid artery who fail to meet evidence-based operative criteria are more than three times as likely to suffer major stroke or death in the next month, when compared to those who do meet those criteria.[11] Thus, it is reasonable to conclude that when scientific, evidence-based medicine is practiced, patients benefit. As such, treatments supported by scientific evidence should be preferred, and scientific evaluation of any treatment that lacks such support should be encouraged.

STANDARDS OF PROOF

Any claim that implies the overthrow of well-established scientific principles has an extraordinary burden of proof. The only rational and practical policy is to ignore extraordinary claims until extraordinary evidence is presented to support them. Anecdotal evidence is ordinary (except in dramatic examples,

---

"Standards of Proof" was written with Victor Stenger, PhD.

such as the use of a defibrillator in cardiac arrest). People can easily be mistaken, tricked, or self-deluded. Placebo-type effects are difficult to eliminate even in the best-designed controlled experiments. Furthermore, a single experiment is never enough; multiple independent replications are essential.

However, not all claims made for CAVM are extraordinary, that is, they would not necessarily violate any established science. For example, some plants may indeed have medicinal benefits, manipulation of a body may help ease its pain, and high-frequency electromagnetic radiation *could* have harmful effects. Still, other claims made by CAVM, if true, would violate well-established science. For example:

- Homeopathic remedies can have an effect beyond placebo.
- The mind can overcome physical laws.
- Health can be improved by manipulating vital energies.

Based on standards of physics, where extraordinary phenomena are often observed, the threshold for publication of extraordinary claims in medical/veterinary journals should be raised considerably, particularly in regards to alternative claims. Most journals in medicine, psychology, and pharmacology allow publication of results at an arbitrarily established significance level of $p = 0.05$ (usually misrepresenting the p value as the probability that the results of the study are valid).[†] However, when a reported effect has a p value of 0.05, it simply means that there is a 1 in 20 chance (5 percent probability) that the results occurred by chance. Statistical significance tests can measure probabilities, but no matter what level of significance is chosen, there is always some probability of seeing a difference between studied groups when none really exists.

Furthermore, p values tell nothing about the clinical significance of an observed effect. Differences may be observed between arms of a study; however, even if those differences are significant, they may not be clinically relevant. For example, studies in the mid-1990s compared the thrombolytic agents streptokinase and tissue plasminogen activator (tPA) to dissolve blood clots in patients post-myocardial infarction. On average, patients receiving tPA gained extra quality days of life, and the difference was highly significant. However, the tPA carried a higher cost and was also associated with a higher incidence of stroke. Thus, when evaluating the overall data, streptokinase was marginally

---

[†]The precise definition of the p value states that if the null hypothesis is correct, then the reported effect of a greater one would occur as a statistical artifact on the average, a fraction p times. That is, the p value makes no statement about the likelihood that the reported effect is real. It only makes a statement about the expected frequency that the effect would result from chance when the effect is not real.

preferred, in spite of the apparent statistical difference in p value.[12] Statistical testing is not a substitute for clinical decision making.

The field of physics is full of examples of extraordinary effects with p values much lower than 0.05 that failed to be replicated and never became part of established knowledge. The accepted criterion for publication in most physics journals is $p = 10^{-4}$. That is, a study is published only when one in ten thousand experiments or a smaller fraction would produce the experimental observation as a statistical artifact. Such a strict threshold would be useful in evaluating extraordinary claims, such as may be made for CAVM. Ordinary claims, consistent with existing science, might be published with weaker significance, with the hope that such reports would do more good than harm.

WARNING FLAGS

In evaluating therapies, one should also be cognizant of red flags that might indicate that a therapy is not scientific. While most claims made for CAVM therapies cannot be supported by good evidence, many other aspects carry hallmarks of pseudoscience.[13] These would include:

1. *Vague, unsupported claims of effectiveness*. Testimonial evidence should be, in general, unpersuasive. For example, a device that advertised, "Leading scientists agree" would not normally be considered scientifically credible, unless the leading scientists and their supporting data were identified.

2. *Misuse of defined scientific terminology*. For example, the discovery of a "unipolar" magnet or magnetic monopole would lead its discoverer to an almost immediate Nobel prize, as magnetic monopoles have not been shown to exist. Similarly, treatments that *detoxify* the body, or *support* the kidneys should be viewed with skepticism, unless such terms and their mechanisms of action were defined.

3. *Mischaracterization of medicine*. It is particularly telling when a therapy tries to distinguish itself from science and medicine. For example, a company might warn about the side effects of taking too many pills, and offer their product as an alternative, while offering no evidence that the product might be effective. Similarly, advocating a treatment as natural or holistic or free of side effects offers little in the way of evidentiary support. Indeed, so-called natural substances are certainly not free of risk (e.g., crotalid venom, poison ivy, etc., etc.); a treatment free of side effects may not have any effects.

4. *Inaccurate claims.* Statements contrary to fact are an indication that a theory is not likely to be clinically useful. For example, one company has stated that studies at various universities have proven that static magnets increase blood flow. This appears to be contrary to fact.

5. *Subjective measurements.* Even though there are times when studies must rely on measurements of subjective experience, subjectivity is notorious for introducing error into results. Objective measurements are ideal; failing such measurements, thorough blinding of evaluators is mandatory.

6. *Ignoring negative results.* Negative results count more against a claim than positive results count for it. This is especially true if negative results continue over time, because if phenomena are real, those studying them should eventually reach the point where they, and eventually, others, can reliably demonstrate it. The steady appearance of treatment failures in the medical literature has been a particular problem for many fields in CAVM, including acupuncture, chiropractic, and homeopathy.

7. *Lack of direct evidence.* Theories should allow themselves to be tested fairly directly. So, for example, if homeopathic molecular patterns are a real phenomenon, those who study homeopathy should be able to demonstrate them.

8. *Predicted phenomena remain slippery.* As experimental and theoretical work progresses, more and more sound evidence for the related phenomena should appear.

9. *No deepening evidence.* Over time, if a clinical effect is useful and relevant, it will become obvious and repeatable. For fields such as chiropractic, acupuncture, and homeopathy, useful clinical effects have remained difficult to establish. Indeed, in spite of hundreds of years of experience and investigation, the state of the art in most alternative therapies appears to have advanced little from the times in which those therapies were initially proposed.

10. *Poor investigation of alternative explanations.* Results claimed for some therapies are often easily explained. For example, opiate rises with acupuncture could also conceivably occur with any form of acupuncture needling—if such rises occur, precise needle placement may not be important. Alternative explanations need to be ruled out before theories are accepted.

11. *Paradigm talk.* A paradigm simply means a philosophical and theoretical framework within which theories, laws, and generalizations, and the experiments performed in support of them, are formulated. When the phrase "paradigm shift" is used to imply a

new theoretical view, such a view prevails in spite of, not because of, good science. For example, the discoverers of quantum mechanics did not have to argue a paradigm shift before their views were accepted—proponents merely presented increasing amounts of good evidence. To the extent that paradigm shift is used to describe social and societal change, it has little legitimate role in discussing the quality of evidence in support of medical treatments. To be considered legitimate, the paradigm shifts of alternative veterinary medicine would seem to require animals to not get anything identifiable, such as diabetes, gastric dilitation and volvulus, Lyme disease, cancer, or other diseases (which they clearly do), and to be adequately treated for anything resembling these conditions using paradigm-specific theory and methodology (which they clearly are not).

12. *Carts before horses.* When there is little evidence to support a belief, proponents of such beliefs tend to offer excuses. Such excuses range from a "lack of funding" to "the medical establishment does not want our therapy to be known." There would be no reason for such excuses if there were good evidence for the beliefs in question. The fact that such excuses are offered is a virtual admission that there is not good evidence to support the beliefs.

ACUPUNCTURE
Human Clinical
Of all of the alternative modalities, acupuncture is perhaps the most exhaustively investigated. Indeed, thousands of acupuncture studies have been conducted. Acupuncture has been assessed in innumerable published comparative human trials involving thousands of patients in a variety of situations, most often for the relief of pain. Unfortunately, most of these trials are handicapped by their poor methodological quality. In addition, studies of the therapeutic usefulness of acupuncture are fraught with methodological difficulties, including the choice of placebo, a suitable control treatment, and the type of stimulation applied. Nevertheless, as of 1999, over 30 years of active acupuncture research failed to unequivocally demonstrate its clinical efficacy in human medicine,[14] and the past several years have not provided indication that would suggest that such demonstrations will be forthcoming.

Controlled trials in human medicine appear to have found evidence of benefit for acupuncture in the treatment of nausea and vomiting, both postoperatively and during pregnancy. Unfortunately, the practical implications of these results are limited, most notably because various unrelated methods were used to stimulate various points (needle insertion, finger pressure, capsicum plaster application, electrical stimulation, etc.). In addition, the success of a variety of unrelated interventions at different points at least suggests that psychological factors—an important component of vomiting in people—are at work. In the positive reports that exist on acupuncture for the prevention of nausea and vomiting, as well as for the treatment of migraine and headache (another condition for which there are some reports of efficacy), researchers have failed to report on important clinical details, rendering readers of such reports unable to critically appraise them from a clinical standpoint. In addition, the design of those reports is such that potential reviewers are unable to establish valid conclusions about the usefulness of acupuncture for such conditions based on the general quality of the design of the studies themselves.[15]

There is certainly no consistency in acupuncture diagnosis or treatment, even when different acupuncturists evaluate the same patient.[16] Also, while some data indicate that acupuncture may be useful for treating headache, neck pain, and low back pain, data are conflicting and no definitive recommendations can be made. For the treatment of addictions, such as alcohol or cocaine dependence, post-stroke rehabilitation, better quality clinical trials fail to demonstrate efficacy for acupuncture.[17] For most of the remaining conditions for which it is used, it is either impossible to draw conclusions about efficacy, or the conclusions are negative.[18,19,20]

In still other areas, such as for surgical anesthesia, the use of acupuncture has been largely abandoned, even in China.[21] Indeed, in light of reports from Chinese surgeons who were forced to operate on human patients given only acupuncture anesthesia, it is difficult to understand why the technique has ever been seriously considered in the West. For example, on October 22, 1980, a report in the Chinese newspaper *Wen-hui-pao* reported the results of over thirty thousand human operations conducted under acupuncture anesthesia. Noting the political pressure on surgeons to use the technique, the authors noted, "If we apply these standards [safety, effectiveness, predictability, etc.] to an assessment of acupuncture anesthesia then, first of all, it cannot achieve absence of pain or basic absence of pain. This is acknowledged in all treatises dealing with acupuncture anesthesia, stated in common language, the suppression of pain is incomplete. . . . The patient undergoes surgery in a state of full consciousness."[22] In addition, given the safety, effectiveness, and reliability of local and general anesthetic techniques, there is good reason to question why acupuncture was ever considered as a realistic option for modern anesthesia.

Veterinary Clinical

Public attention has been focused on acupuncture as a possible therapeutic intervention for animals by the media, and veterinary interest has arisen from books and publications on the subject. Interest in acupuncture from the veterinary profession has been primarily driven by owner demand and practitioner curiosity. However, evidence of the clinical efficacy of acupuncture from scientific trials in treating any clinical condition in any animal species is virtually nonexistent;[23] instead, most veterinary studies on acupuncture are reported as case series.

The veterinary literature is remarkable for the number of conditions in which acupuncture use has been reported, but just as remarkable in that virtually all of those reports are based on uncontrolled observations. This fact often results in a disparity between published information and clinical studies; for example, whereas animal acupuncture has been advocated in pain management,[24] controlled trials in dogs[25] and horses[26] have not supported its use. Similarly, while acupuncture may be recommended for the treatment of canine epilepsy,[27] no controlled veterinary trials appear to exist, and acupuncture fails to show either a clinical effect[28] or an effect on health-related quality of life in epilepsy[29] in humans.

Much research on acupuncture in animals pertains to pain modulation. Effects, when they can be shown, most likely only represent short-term hypalgesia, which is most likely brought about by the mechanisms behind stress-induced analgesia and the activation of diffuse noxious inhibitory control. In addition, virtually all of the experimental acupuncture research has been performed with electroacupuncture even though the prescribed therapeutic applications of acupuncture are generally manual.[30] It is entirely reasonable, therefore, to consider that such effects as occur due to electroacupuncture are electrical rather than acupuncture related and may not require precise placement of needles at all, even if those effects do have clinical relevance.

The only attempt at a systematic review of acupuncture completed in animals to date, in horses, found that the equine acupuncture literature does not focus on quantitative analyses and rarely fits any of the relevant criteria considered necessary for a good scientific investigation. That is, such protocols as randomization, blinding, control groups, and other typical aspects of quality studies are lacking in virtually every published paper in the field. Nevertheless, a few individual equine studies meet some standards for good scientific investigation, although these standards vary greatly among the papers. However, in general, equine acupuncture studies are quite small and vary in their endpoints (making a pooling of results impossible). As in small animals, almost none of the studies that meet selection criteria evaluate filiform-needle acupuncture; rather, they look at electrical stimulation, hormonal responses to needling, or the effects of drugs placed at putative acupuncture points. With those caveats, the review concluded that the equine acupuncture literature conducted under generally accepted criteria for good-quality scientific investigations does not favor the use of this technique. Nor do such good-quality papers as exist provide consistent results when studies have been conducted attempting to replicate previously obtained data.[31] No reviews of the efficacy of small animal acupuncture appear to have been conducted.

In general, veterinary acupuncture studies are poorly designed, a fact that is consistent with evaluations of other alternative modalities in human medicine.[32] There are exceptions; however, in general, the best studies are least likely to show positive results. Thus, there is at least the possibility that erroneous conclusions can be drawn about the value of animal acupuncture from taking such positive studies or reports as exist on its success at face value.

Points and Meridians

Research on the nature of acupuncture points and the channels along which those points are supposedly connected (meridians) is often difficult to evaluate because of the diverse nature of the claims made, incomplete data provided in published studies, and the variety of parameters involved in the assessment of these claims. However, neither acupuncture points nor meridians have been shown to exist. Obvious contradictions exist between current acupuncture practice and those described in the historical record.[33] In addition, there appears to be little agreement on the correct number of points and meridians among modern practitioners of acupuncture (veterinary or human). Furthermore, if one traces the historical record, points and meridians have moved repeatedly over the centuries (that is, different sources show different points, as well as numbers and placement of meridians).

Acupuncture points may sometimes be located in the vicinity of peripheral nerves, ligaments, or tendons.[34] However, there is no consistent association with any one specific gross anatomical structure in any species. Several investigators have reported various histological findings at acupuncture points, such as nerve terminals, neurovascular bundles, or mast cell accumulations; however, none of the studies has used statistical evaluation of quantitative histological data.[35]

No method of determining acupuncture point locations has been shown to be precise or repeatable. Electrical skin resistance, which can be detected by various devices, has been shown to be an inaccurate method of locating acupuncture points and is influenced by such factors as the shape and surface area of the electrode, the dryness of the skin, the inclination of the electrode, the electrode gel used, the scanning speed of the device, and even room temperature and humidity.[36,37,38,39,40] Traditional methods of acupuncture point location in humans rely on the *cun* unit, said to be equal to the width of the interphalangeal joint of the human thumb. However, this method, subject to individual anatomic variation, has been shown to be unreliable.[41] Acupuncture points have failed to demonstrate sensitivity to palpation relative to other points on the human body; its value as the sole form of point location is doubtful.[42] Finally, directional and proportional methods for measuring acupuncture point locations—the most widely used methods for locating acupuncture points in humans—have also been shown to be grossly imprecise.[43] Accordingly, even Felix Mann, a cofounder of the British Acupuncture Society, has concluded that acupuncture points do not exist and has observed that, if modern human acupuncture texts are to be believed, there is no skin left that is not an acupuncture point.[44]

Further muddying the empirical waters is the fact that some types of acupuncture in human medicine do not use a traditional theoretical basis. In these approaches (e.g., Western acupuncture), needle placement may be unrelated to the presence or absence of actual anatomical acupuncture point entities. The irrelevance of specific points for any effects of acupuncture is underscored by the fact that most studies that have compared sham and real acupuncture points have been unable to show a consistent difference in response to manipulation between sites;[45] similar efficacy has been asserted between traditional and transpositional points in horses.[46]

From a pragmatic standpoint, one might surmise that if such structures as acupuncture points and meridians did exist and could be reliably demonstrated, they would revolutionize the study of anatomy and physiology; however, no such revolutions have been forthcoming to date. Whatever the clinical efficacy of needling, there is, as yet, no compelling evidence to show that acupuncture points or meridians exist as discrete entities.[47,48]

Mechanism of Action

It should come as no surprise to anyone with an education in basic physiology that inserting needles into a body will invoke some sort of a physiologic response. Indeed, most animal studies have demonstrated *some* physiologic effect of needling, although the clinical relevance of such effects remains questionable. In humans, functional MRI studies, which measure increased oxygen uptake in areas of the brain, have suggested that the brain is aware when a needle has been placed in the body, but fail to demonstrate that this response is specific to the areas stimulated with acupuncture needles or consistent correlations between the points selected and the areas of the cerebral cortex that are purportedly associated with those points.[49,50] The erythema and inflammation that result from needle insertion are not unique to acupuncture points, and human patients report identical sensations whether real or sham acupuncture points are used.[51] The distribution of the effects of acupuncture on pressure pain threshold does not support either neural, segmental, or traditional Chinese medicine channel theories, and needling nonacupoints leads to statistically significant increases in pain pressure threshold at six sites when needles are manipulated.[52] Finally, identical, transient, quick reflex responses of the sympathetic nervous system have been seen whether real or sham points are needled.[53]

Purported scientific mechanisms of action for acupuncture generally involve suggestions that the procedure elevates circulating levels of various neurochemicals, especially endorphins (endogenous opiates). While elevations in endorphins certainly are associated with some acupuncture investigations, such an explanation is not convincing. Endorphins have a very short half-life and should not be responsible for the prolonged effects claimed by acupuncture proponents; endorphin levels in human serum have a half-life of around 22 minutes;[54] endorphins in the human central nervous system persist for approximately 317 minutes.[55] Furthermore, fine-needle acupuncture is not associated with rises in central nervous system endorphins in horses.[56] Further confusing the picture is the fact that endorphins may rise due to any number of stimuli; even running and shipping elevate plasma endorphins in horses.[57] Endorphins are also credited for placebo analgesia responses.[58] Nor do other purported hormonal rises attributed to acupuncture appear to be significant; for example, plasma cortisol has been shown to both increase[59] and decrease[60] after acupuncture in the horse.

Numerous plausible—and simpler—explanations for the effects of acupuncture exist, including expectation,[61] suggestion, counterirritation,[62] and operant conditioning, as well as the diffuse noxious inhibitory stimulus (whereby a noxious stimulus at one site interferes with the perception of pain at another site).[63] Indeed, as pertains to the diffuse noxious inhibitory stimulus, while one study found that acupuncture suppressed the pain response to a cutaneous prick or electrical stimulation of a rat's tail, the most effective suppression was obtained by a simple pinch.[64]

Other potential mechanisms of action of acupuncture-related therapies are perhaps not so surprising. For example, electroacupuncture has been shown to provide mild rectal analgesia in an experimental model in horses, although less than what was provided by the drug butorphanol.[65] However, there is absolutely no reason to believe that the effects seen have anything to do with acupuncture, given that precise needle placement was not shown to be important (that is, the study lacked a sham control) and that electrical stimulation was involved. Indeed, such therapies as transcutaneous electrical nerve stimulation (TENS) employ electricity for pain management[66] (albeit with conflicting results). Indeed, there is reason to doubt that even needle skin penetration is important when using electrical stimuli in efforts to control pain; variants of electroacupuncture exist using skin patch electrodes, and identical clinical effectiveness is claimed.[67]

Acupuncture Diagnostics

Palpation of putative acupuncture points has also been used diagnostically. Such diagnostic attempts have not stood up to scrutiny. In humans, palpation of a particular acupuncture point on the right leg was not useful in the diagnosis of appendicitis,[68] and palpation of the point considered most diagnostic for equine protozoal myelitis was considered poor when compared with that by conventional diagnostic methods.[69]

Safety

The complications of acupuncture, although infrequent, cannot be overlooked. In humans, reported complications include infections (mainly hepatitis), and organ, tissue, and nerve injury.[70] Adverse effects in humans include cutaneous disorders,[71] hypotension, fainting, and vomiting.[72] Complications can occasionally be severe, especially regarding infections related to nonsterile needles and pneumothorax. However, most of these risks might be avoided by the use of more rigorous techniques and, in general, the risks of acupuncture do not appear to be considerable.[73] In animals, adverse events are largely unreported, although one might easily imagine that some animals would resent the insertion of needles into various locations on their bodies.

CHIROPRACTIC

Human

The current state of basic scientific knowledge concerning the elusive subluxation (or, vertebral subluxation complex [VSC] as it may be more generally described by some) can be summed up as, "There is now sufficient scientific investigation to develop working models to explain the effects of the adjustment. However, there is insufficient evidence to state that any particular theory can be considered valid."[74] Unfortunately, in chiropractic literature, the lack of current knowledge tends to be extrapolated into speculation and chiropractic theories may be presented as fact. In fact, there is inadequate basic science data to substantiate the existence of the VSC, and there are few (if any) randomized, controlled, clinical trials of spinal manipulation that have monitored presumed indicators of the putative VSC. Therefore, it is not appropriate to claim that by manipulating the VSC, a therapeutic benefit in humans or animals can be achieved.[75] Furthermore, even if such lesions could be shown to exist in the human spine, the commonly used diagnostic measures to detect them are neither reproducible nor reliable.[76,77]

Although there are several dozen randomized, controlled trials (RCTs) supporting an analgesic and mobility-restoring benefit of manipulation for human patients with low back pain and related musculoskeletal conditions,[78,79] systematic reviews and meta-analyses conducted during the 1990s made cautiously positive or equivocal statements about the effectiveness of manipulation for its various applications.[80,81,82,83,84] This is because, overall, the quality of the studies and the reviews was not good.[85] Furthermore, even when clinical efficacy has been shown statistically, it is generally of marginal value clinically, and benefits typically depend on specific points in time at which the observations were made.[86]

It is important to note that trials supporting manipulation for the relief of back pain are not restricted to chiropractic manipulations; many different providers may perform various manipulations, many of which have nothing to do with subluxations. However, a 2001 review of sham-controlled, double-blind, randomized clinical trials on spinal manipulation, suggested that spinal manipulation was not associated with clinically relevant therapeutic effects.[87] Indeed, in most of the RCTs of manipulation for musculoskeletal pain, the positive effects noted tend to be statistically significant but not dramatic or even clinically relevant. Other studies have shown that manipulative interventions may not be better than minimal intervention provided by an educational booklet on how to take care of a sore back.[88] In terms of long-term outcomes, chiropractic has not been shown to have benefit when compared to other treatments for studied conditions. Although chiropractors may recommend their therapies for conditions not related to the musculoskeletal system, reviews of chiropractic treatment of conditions not related to the musculoskeletal system have not shown benefit.[89,90] Thus, to summarize, the research to date has shown that spinal manipulation may be effective only in a narrow subset of human patients, and in these patients, it is no more effective than other treatments.[91,92] The mechanism(s) of such therapeutic effects as occur from manipulative therapy have not been established. Many of the traditional, segmental indicators of the VSC have failed to demonstrate reproducibility (interexaminer reliability) among clinicians.[93,94] None of the presumed indicators of VSC has been shown to predict illness (i.e., symptoms, altered physiological function), nor has their eradication (by manipulation) been shown to confer clinical benefit. No particular form of manipulative therapy has been shown to be superior to another. That is, there is no evidence that chiropractic manipulations are of more benefit than maneuvers that may be performed by other practitioners, including osteopaths, or physical therapists.

Dozens of chiropractic maneuvers and techniques exist and there has been much discussion and dissension about their relative merits.[95,96] Chiropractors' manual methods have diverse origins, coming both from within and outside of the chiropractic field. Optimum technique has been a source of controversy within the field, but virtually nothing has been done to determine the relative merits of various manual assessment and intervention procedures. There is also much question about what methods are used; the proprietary nature of many chiropractic methods has promoted both innovation and secrecy.[97] Furthermore, chiropractors have not confined themselves to the adjustive procedures that marked the profession's inception. They tend to add various other physical modalities, such as heat and cold, to their manipulations, although these interventions have been shown to be of no benefit beyond manipulations alone.[98]

The types of clinical research that would be required to create a gold-standard for the VSC have been discussed;[99] reasons for complacency in VSC-related research have also been suggested.[100,101] However, in short, the clinical evidence for the meaningfulness/utility of the VSC is barely more than anecdotal and a century of anecdotes has yet to give rise to experimental proof of the traditional chiropractic lesion. In addition, the overall utility of manipulative therapy for the treatment of musculoskeletal pain has not been established. As such, as of 2003, several of the states of the United States of America, including Massachusetts, Vermont, California, Indiana, Michigan, Minnesota, New Hampshire, New Jersey, Ohio, and Texas, have either cut or have proposed cutting government funding for chiropractic services.[102]

There is no consensus within the chiropractic profession on what chiropractic is or should be. As proposed by its founder, chiropractic was a panacea for all diseases based on the correction of impinged spinal nerves that could be corrected by spinal adjustment. Many chiropractors have moved away from this definition, but there is much division within the chiropractic profession about the scope of practice (e.g., should chiropractic be limited to musculoskeletal problems in the way that podiatrists limit themselves to feet or dentists to teeth? Are chiropractors primary care providers? Should chiropractors treat animals?).

Finally, even as the scientific deficiencies of chiropractic are pointed out, the chiropractic profession appears to be entrenched in nonscientific and antiscientific messages. The largest professional associations in the United States and Canada routinely distribute patient brochures that make claims for chiropractic that cannot be currently justified by available scientific evidence or that are intrinsically untestable. These assertions simply reinforce the image of the chiropractic profession as one that operates outside the boundaries of science.[103]

Mechanism of Action

Chiropractors assert that they direct spinal manipulations at specific dysfunctional joints (curiously, when other, nonspinal joints are dysfunctional, manipulation is generally not considered). Typically, this dysfunction is characterized as a form of joint sprain or strain, with associated descriptive terms such as *hypomobility*, *malalignment*, or *muscle tension*, among others.[104] Chiropractic theory has held that attention to these problems via "adjustment" can have important physiologic effects, such as increased range of joint motion,[105,106] changes in kinematics of vertebral facet joints,[107] increased tolerance for pain,[108] and changes in endorphin levels[109] among others.

However, subluxation of a vertebra, as originally defined by chiropractic, and involving the exertion of pressure on spinal nerves, does not occur, regardless of which theory is subscribed to.[110] In addition, recent work has suggested that the concept of specific, directed manipulations is untenable. During a chiropractic manipulation, the effective loading of specific target sites of individual vertebrae or spinal segments is much smaller than the global measures of total force applied might suggest; that is, the total force applied to a particular area is not the same as the total force applied to the body. This is because as the forces during spinal manipulative treatment increase, so does the contact area; therefore, much of the total treatment force is taken up by non-target-specific tissues. Such dissipation of forces would be expected to be even more dramatic in larger animals, such as horses. Thus, it appears that, to the extent that spinal manipulative treatments have been successful, it is not because of the precisely directed and amplitude-controlled force (which seems impossible) but despite the fact that these forces cannot be applied precisely.[111]

Safety

The safety of spinal manipulation has been the subject of considerable controversy in the human field. The risk of serious complications from lumbar manipulations appears to be quite low.[112] However, cervical manipulations have been associated with the risk of serious, even fatal, cerebrovascular accidents,[113] although the frequency of such complications is the subject of discussion.[114] Regardless, it is not reasonable to rely on reports of harm as an accurate estimate of harm—calculating the number of serious accidents caused by neck manipulation simply by counting the cases reported in medical journals is as valid as calculating the number of victims of traffic accidents by reading only the same medical journals. *No* risk of treatment is acceptable if there is no accompanying therapeutic benefit.

Veterinary Manual Therapy (Veterinary Chiropractic)

From a mechanical standpoint, it should be obvious that the forces on the spine of an animal that walks on four limbs are quite different from those of humans, who walk on two. Thus, even if human chiropractic theories were plausible, direct application of those theories to animals might not be warranted. There are additional mechanical considerations, for example, since the vertebrae of horses are the size of the adult fist and surrounded by muscle, tendon, and ligament layers several inches thick, it seems reasonable to wonder whether equine vertebrae can actually be manipulated.

It may be reasonable to surmise that moving an animal's limbs around, massaging its muscles, or giving it any sort of attention might be well received by the animal, but there is no evidence that such attention can improve health. Apparently, no controlled experimental research of the clinical effects of adjusting animals has been published to date. There are no systematic, prospective, controlled outcome data to substantiate a beneficial effect of musculoskeletal manipulation of animals. Furthermore, no published study has ever shown how a chiropractic-related problem can be diagnosed in animals or even how treatment success is determined.

HOMEOPATHY

Human

Several reviews and meta-analyses of homeopathy have been performed over the past approximately 20 years. There have been at least four meta-analyses and six reviews of the effects of homeopathic medications in human patients.

A 1990 review of 40 published randomized trials of homeopathy in human medicine found that most of the studies had major methodological flaws and concluded that, "the results do not provide acceptable evidence that homeopathic treatments are effective."[115]

A 1991 meta-analysis of homeopathy in human medicine concluded, "At the moment the evidence of clinical trials is positive but not sufficient to draw definitive conclusions because most trials are of low methodological quality and because of the unknown role of publication bias. This indicates that there is a legitimate case for further evaluation of homeopathy, but only by means of well performed trials." The investigators also noted that, "Critical people who do not believe in the efficacy of homeopathy before reading the evidence presented here probably will still not be convinced; people who were more ambivalent in advance will perhaps have a more optimistic view now, whereas people who already believed in the efficacy of homeopathy might at this moment be almost certain that homeopathy works."[116] In a later letter, the authors noted that, "The results of our review would probably be interpreted differently if laboratory studies showed convincing evidence that there is some action of high potencies."[117]

A 1992 German review of homeopathy concluded that, "due to the advance of alternative medicine, a critical synopsis by means of the comparison between scientific medicine (clinical medicine) and homeopathy is warranted. The review of studies carried out according to current scientific criteria revealed—at best—a placebo effect of homeopathy. Until now there is no proven mechanism for the mode of action of homeopathy. Sometimes so-called 'alternative medicine' prevents effective curative measures. In spite of the justified criticism concerning the technical overestimation of classical medicine, scientific research should remain the basis of clinical work."[118]

A 1994 review and meta-analysis of serial agitated dilutions (SAD) in experimental toxicology stated that, "as with clinical studies, the overall quality of toxicology research using SAD preparations is low. The majority of studies either could not be reevaluated by the reviewers or were of such low quality that their likelihood of validity is doubtful. The number of methodologically sound, independently reproduced studies is too small to make any definitive conclusions regarding the effect of SAD preparations in toxicology."[119]

A 1996 review of homeopathy concluded that

- No one should ignore the role of nonspecific factors in therapeutic efficacy, such as the natural history of a given disease and the placebo effect. Indeed, these factors can be used to therapeutic advantage.
- As homeopathic treatments are generally used in conditions with variable outcome or showing spontaneous recovery (hence their placebo responsiveness), these treatments are widely considered to have an effect in some patients.
- However, despite the large number of comparative trials carried out to date, there is no evidence that homeopathy is any more effective than placebo therapy given in identical conditions.
- We believe that homeopathic preparations should not be used to treat serious diseases when other drugs are known to be both effective and safe.
- Pending further evidence, homeopathy remains a form of placebo therapy.[120]

A 1997 meta-analysis concluded, "The results of our meta-analysis are not compatible with the hypothesis that the clinical effects of homeopathy are completely due to placebo. However, we found insufficient evidence from these studies that homeopathy is clearly efficacious for any single clinical condition." Furthermore, "our study has no major implications for clinical practice because we found little evidence of effectiveness of any single homeopathic approach on any single clinical condition." The authors concluded by calling for more research, "providing it is rigorous and systematic."[121] One critic of the study cautioned that when the best trials were examined, the odds of a positive effect of the therapy were distinctly lower than in the overall study.[122] Another critic suggested further caution in interpreting the results of this study by noting that negative trials may have been less likely to be published, which may have skewed the analysis.[123] Finally, in a later study, the lead author himself noted in a later analysis, which evaluated study quality on outcome in placebo-controlled trials of homeopathy, that his original study "at least overestimated the effects of homeopathic treatments."[124]

Another meta-analysis conducted in 1997 examined the use of homeopathy for the treatment of postoperative ileus, measured by the time to first flatus. The investigators concluded that their analyses "do not provide evidence for the use of a particular homeopathic remedy or for a combination of remedies for postoperative ileus. Several drawbacks inherent in the original studies and in the methodology of meta-analysis preclude a firm conclusion." Given those caveats, the study also suggested that homeopathic dilutions less than 12C, those that may contain some of the original substance, had a significant effect, whereas dilutions greater than 12C, which are so dilute as to contain none of the original substance, had none.[125]

In 1999, a systematic review of 120 preclinical investigations of homeopathy was conducted. The author found that lack of independent replication, severe methodological flaws, and contradictory results precluded any firm conclusion. Nevertheless, the review casts great doubt on one of the main assumptions of homeopathy, that is, that extremely diluted homeopathic remedies have biological activity.[126]

A 2002 systematic review of all of the systematic reviews of homeopathy concluded that published research does not support the use of homeopathic products. After 11 previous reviews were evaluated, the article concluded:

> Collectively they failed to provide strong evidence in favour of homeopathy. In particular, there was no condition which responds convincingly better to homeopathic treatment than to placebo or other control interventions. Similarly, there was no homeopathic remedy that was demonstrated to yield clinical effects that are convincingly different from placebo. It is concluded that the best clinical evidence for homeopathy available to date does not warrant positive recommendations for its use in clinical practice.[127]

Finally, and consistent with the previous findings, a 2003 critical overview of homeopathy in human medicine concludes that homeopathy should not be substituted for proven therapies.[128]

Randomized, placebo-controlled, double-blind studies have shown homeopathic remedies to be ineffective in the treatment of adenoid vegetations in children,[129] for control of pain and infection after total abdominal hysterectomy,[130] for prophylaxis of migraine headache,[131,132] and for prevention of pain and bruising following hand surgery.[133] Nor did the effect of homeopathic treatment on mental symptoms of patients with generalized anxiety disorder differ from that of placebo.[134] To date, no single study of homeopathy showing positive results has been successfully replicated. Furthermore, a large study refuted previously obtained results that homeopathic immunotherapy was effective in the treatment of patients with asthma related to allergies to house-dust mites.[135]

Finally, negative homeopathic outcomes have been criticized based on the claim that the treatments used were not based on classical homeopathy, that is, that the treatments were not individualized for each patient. While such criticisms may be considered self-serving in light of the fact that homeopathic remedies are freely available in absence of such considerations, studies evaluating individualized homeopathy have been conducted, as well. So, for example, adjunctive homeopathic remedies, as prescribed by experienced homeopathic practitioners, were no different from placebo in improving the quality of life of children with mild to moderate asthma in addition to conventional treatment in primary care.[136]

Curiously, the lack of good evidence of effectiveness of homeopathic remedies may be irrelevant to supporters of homeopathy. One leading advocate has asserted that proving the effectiveness of homeopathy through scientific research is not important and suggests that personal experience is more important than any number of carefully controlled studies.[137] The importance of personal experience should be considered in light of the fact that positive expectations and beliefs of patients and their doctors historically resulted in reports of excellent or good outcomes in more than 70 percent of cases for the unrelated treatments of five studied conditions, even though the treatments given are now known to have been worthless.[138]

Mechanism of Action

No known, or even credible, mechanism of action by which extremely dilute homeopathic preparations might have a therapeutic effect exists. Further doubt on the significance of homeopathic provings has been cast due to more recent controlled studies in which healthy subjects reported similar symptoms whether given a homeopathic dilution or a placebo.[139,140,141] Indeed, no study has been able to distinguish homeopathic remedies from control solutions, by any method of analysis.

Safety

It is generally conceded that homeopathic remedies are largely safe, especially at high dilutions. Such a finding would not be unexpected were the remedy to contain only a water and/or alcohol solvent (that is, that the solution would contain none of the original substance).

However, while infrequent, there are reports of adverse reactions to homeopathic medications in human patients. Adverse reactions have been reported ranging from pruritus and a measleslike skin rash to anaphylactic shock,[142] pancreatitis,[143] and contact dermatitis.[144] In regard to the safety of homeopathic remedies, the previously cited 1996 review stated,

> Serious adverse effects have been reported with low dilutions (<4C) given parenterally or orally. However, high dilutions (>5C) administered orally or sublingually appear to be entirely safe. We believe that homeopathic preparations should not be used to treat serious diseases when other drugs are known to be both effective and safe. In addition, regardless of the condition treated, dilution below 5CH

(e.g., 3 or 4CH and especially decimal dilutions or mother tinctures) must not only be considered as having no proven efficacy but also as having potential dangers.

Homeopathy and Vaccination

Further concerns regarding safety of homeopathic philosophy and practice arise from the apparent attitude against immunization voiced by some practitioners of homeopathy. In human medicine, several surveys have demonstrated that homeopathic practitioners routinely advise their clients against immunization.[145,146,147,148] The origin of homeopathic antipathy to vaccination is unknown; there is nothing in Hahnemann's writings against immunization.[149] It may arise from a general hostility toward modern medicine that, according to studies, appears to be prevalent within complementary medicine in general.[150]

Homeopathic practitioners may also employ "homeopathic vaccines" or "nosodes" prepared from high dilutions of infectious agents, material such as vomitus, discharges, fecal matter, or infected tissues. Curiously, nosodes are not prepared according to homeopathic principles; rather, they would be more properly described as being isopathy (that is, preparations obtained from diseased material). Samuel Hahnemann himself decried the use of such preparations[151] and was a supporter of smallpox vaccination.[152]

There is no evidence at all to suggest that homeopathic immunizations have any effectiveness.[153] To the contrary, there is one case reported in the human literature where a patient followed her homeopath's advice and took a homeopathic immunization against malaria before traveling to an endemic area. The patient promptly got malaria.[154] It is of note that the British Faculty of Homeopathy acknowledges the effectiveness of vaccines and recommends their use in humans.[155]

Veterinary Homeopathy

At least three reviews of veterinary homeopathy have been published. In 1985, a chapter on veterinary homeopathy concluded,

> Contrary to what you hear or read too often, rigorous scientific demonstration of the therapeutic effect of homeopathic remedies in veterinary medicine has not yet been done. Although it may seem exaggerated to conclude that homeopathy has absolutely no place, from a pragmatic point of view, in veterinary medicine, it is obvious that future works will have to bend to the new modern methodologies in order to be able to take away the firm beliefs of stern minds.[156]

A 1993 German review of homeopathy in veterinary medicine offered several conclusions:

- Doctor and veterinarian are similarly obligated to apply the therapeutic measure that prevailing opinions deem most effective.
  Where there is for particular definite illnesses a particularly effective and generally recognized treatment, in such cases the supporters of homeopathy may not disregard the better successes
  from their own differing direction.
- It is undisputed that homeopathy in the area of stronger potency
  can achieve effects pharmacologically and toxicologically; the
  superiority of homeopathy as a therapeutic measure in comparison with conventional therapy methods is at this point not verified. Moreover, the harmlessness of homeopathy in stronger
  potency is for the most part not verified.
- The effectiveness of homeopathy in middle and high potencies is
  up to now not verified. It is undisputed that with the help of
  homeopathy, not insignificant placebo effects can be achieved. In
  veterinary medicine, giving an animal an "active" placebo and
  another a "passive" can play a significant role and influence the
  owner.[157]

A 1998 review of homeopathic treatment in animals suggested approaching homeopathy with an "open mind."[158] As evidence for the effectiveness of
homeopathic treatment in animals, the study cites three studies in which
some clinical evidence of effectiveness was seen, seven in which the results
were difficult to interpret for various reasons, and six in which there was
either no response to treatment or worsening of the condition. Several of the
studies cited were performed on healthy animals. In one of the studies in
which the condition of sick animals worsened, the worsening of the animals'
health was taken as possible evidence of treatment effectiveness, according to
Herring's law. (Critics would note that such a law or healing crisis would
mean that one cannot lose when administering homeopathic medications
because whether the patient improves or gets worse, the treatment may be
viewed as being successful.)

Very few of the animal and in vitro studies on homeopathy have been rigorously conducted. Most studies have not been properly blinded nor randomized and small numbers of animals have been used. However, one high-quality
study was unable to distinguish between a commercially available homeopathic remedy and placebo for the treatment of canine atopic dermatitis[159] and
another double-blind randomized placebo controlled trial on homeopathic
treatment of neonatal calf diarrhea, comprising 44 calves in 12 dairy herds,
showed no clinical statistical difference between groups (the placebo group
actually had a slightly shorter duration of diarrhea).[160]

Experiments comparing high-dilution homeopathic preparations to both a placebo group and a known effective treatment group are largely absent, as are studies with predefined outcome variables. In addition, researchers have been guilty of not reporting differences (if such existed) between the homeopathy and placebo groups. While the animals (and tissue preparations) may not be susceptible to suggestibility, clearly the researcher making the critical observations could be influenced. It is useful to consider that animals may respond to any changes in their environment, which could also be confused with a response to homeopathic medication.[161]

Nosodes in Veterinary Medicine

Homeopathic nosodes have failed to protect dogs from death due to parvoviral enteritis[162] and calves from parasitic bronchitis caused by *Dictyocaulus viviparus*.[163] Notwithstanding legitimate concerns regarding the safety of immunization in animals, it seems inconceivable that an ethical veterinary practitioner would ever recommend against the use of proven effective vaccine prophylaxis, most particularly in the case of diseases such as rabies, in which there is potential for transmission to humans. Nosodes will appear to be highly effective as long as the majority of animals remains vaccinated. However, if the use of such agents were to become widespread, as soon as a nonvaccinated animal population is large enough to allow virulent agents to spread, disease outbreaks would likely occur, returning veterinary medicine to where it was decades ago.[164]

HERBALS AND BOTANICALS

Human

Historical Evidence

Although the long history of the use of herbal and botanical products may suggest to some that such products are effective medicines, a more critical look reveals some significant difficulties with such a preconception. By historical standards, herbal and botanical medicines were not responsible for any measurable improvement in human health. Prior to the advent of modern pharmacology in the twentieth century, life was, to quote Thomas Hobbes (1588–1679), "poor, nasty, brutish and short." Mortality curves for nineteenth-century cities were largely identical to those of preagrarian societies and death rates spiked during years of infectious epidemics. The high morbidity and short life spans in prescientific societies were due, at least in part, to the inability to treat infectious diseases, which points to the general inefficacy of herbal therapies. In a forty-thousand-year-old Paleolithic society in Morocco, examination of skeletons shows that 50 percent of the population died before age 38. Mortality curves remained surprisingly similar over thousands of subsequent years and under diverse cultural conditions.[165] In 1900, life expectancy was 45 years; however, in 1996 it was 76.1 years. These dramatic changes were largely due to clean water, vaccination, and the ability to control infections via pharmacology.[166]

When discussing the historical efficacy of herbal medications, one must also ask the question "Effective compared to what?" Medical treatments available at the time of wide herbal use, such as bleeding, or prescribing large doses of mercury salts, were largely ineffective. As with homeopathy, the use of a botanical product that lacked acute toxicity might be expected to be of less harm to the patient than other therapeutic interventions. Furthermore, the wide historical use of herbal medications may also be due to the fact that conventional health care was not affordable for or available to much of the population.

Historical assessments of herbal therapies must also be made in light of vast differences between historical and current use of the products. In the past, the emphasis for their use was on treatment of symptoms, rather than underlying disease conditions (which had yet to be identified). Elimination of the symptom, rather than elimination of the underlying problem, was the criterion used for treatment success. For example, if a fever abated due to ingesting willow bark, the treatment would have worked, although the disease process that caused the fever might have been unaffected. In addition, herbal and botanical remedies were generally applied for vague, all-encompassing conditions (e.g., liver malfunction). Again, such prescriptions should not be surprising in light of the fact that the remedies were prescribed in an era when disease etiology was uncertain, when different diseases with the same symptoms could not be differentiated, and where the physician had few tools to work with. However, the nature of the claims made for efficacy, the uncertain identities of the plants actually used, and the vague nature of the conditions treated makes it exceedingly difficult to objectively evaluate the true utility of the remedies employed.

Scientific Evidence

Herbal medicines (defined here as preparations derived from plants and fungi, either as crude products or, for example, by alcoholic extraction or decoction, which are used to prevent and treat diseases) are an important component of traditional medicine in virtually every culture.[167] In other countries, herbal and botanical products are an important market. For example, Germany has a long tradition in the use of herbal preparations marketed as drugs. In the United States and the United Kingdom, herbal medicinal products are marketed as food supplements or botanical medicines. Traditional healers in the Third World commonly employ herbs.[168]

A considerable number of systematic reviews on herbal medicines are available, however, only a relative few of the medicinal plants that may be employed in herbal therapies have been tested in controlled trials, which, no matter how promising the laboratory experiments or anecdotal experiences reported, are required. One good example of the failure of anecdote is highlighted by a trial in which a mistletoe extract, which was reputed to have anticancer properties and has shown some interesting properties in in vitro research, did not affect disease-free survival or the quality of life in human patients with cancer of the head and neck.[169]

In the majority of instances, reviewers of herbal medicines considered the available evidence as promising but only very rarely as convincing and sufficient as a firm basis for clinical decisions. Many reviewers have criticized the methodological quality of the primary studies.[170] Trials using firm endpoints are very rarely available and periods of observation are usually short. The clinical relevance of the observed effects is not always clear. The reviews mostly show that the reported effects of herbal products are rather limited, need further confirmation by well-designed trials, or both. In addition, data that directly compare herbal remedies with well-established pharmaceutical products are often not available or do not provide much useful information (for example, data may be derived from studies that failed to include a placebo group).[171]

Herbal medicinal products are not, in general, subject to patent protection. Thus, drug companies may not be motivated to invest in trials of crude plant preparations (although drug companies routinely engage in large-scale pharmacological screening of herbs). Instead, many of the existing herbal medicine manufacturers are comparatively small companies. Perhaps this may help explain why the quality of many herbal medicine trials is low. However, it is also reasonable to consider that negative trials, which could threaten the company's survival, might not be published.

A basic problem concerning all clinical research in herbal medicines is the question of whether different products, extracts, or even different lots of the same extract are comparable and equivalent. Quality assurance is necessary to ensure that a particular herbal product has the expected effect; it is also an important determinant of product safety. For example, echinacea products may contain other plant extracts, use different plant species (*E. purpurea, pallida*, or *angustifolia*) and different parts (herb, root, both), and might have been produced in quite different manners (hydro- or lipophilic extraction). In addition, the concentration of active ingredients can vary dramatically depending on where the plants were grown or when they were harvested.[172] Finally, even a claim of standardization does not mean the preparation is accurately labeled, nor does it indicate less variability in concentration of constituents of the herb.[173] Thus, it may not be possible to extrapolate the results of any one study to any particular product.

In short, systematic reviews are often a good tool to get an overview of available evidence from clinical trials of individual herbal preparations used in people. In addition, some herbal and botanical remedies may have pharmacological effects. However, applying the findings of individual trials in human medicine to animal patients' care is problematic, for many reasons.

Mechanism(s) of Action

In the laboratory, plant extracts have been shown to have a variety of pharmacological effects, including anti-inflammatory, vasodilatory, antimicrobial, anticonvulsant, sedative, and antipyretic effects. This should not be surprising, as many plants contain pharmacologically active ingredients, many of which appear to be produced as a defense mechanism for the plants. For example, one important subset of natural chemicals includes plant toxins that appear to protect plants against fungi, insects, and animal predators. Thousands of such compounds are known, and individual species may contain a few dozen toxins, including numerous carcinogens and mutagens.[174] Such compounds are certainly not benign. For example, kava kava, which has been advocated for the treatment of anxiety, depression, and insomnia in humans, is also hepatotoxic.[175] In addition, some abnormal laboratory test results and toxic effects are seen in humans due to the use of herbal medicines.[343] While toxicity of a particular compound is certainly dose dependent, so is pharmacologic activity, and, accordingly, so is the medical clinical relevance of such activity.

Method of Prescription

Although superficially similar, herbal medicine and conventional pharmacotherapy may have three important differences.

1. *Use of whole plants.* Herbalists often use unpurified plant extracts containing several different constituents. They may claim that these can work together synergistically so that the effect of the whole herb is greater than the summed effects of its components. They also may claim that toxicity is reduced when whole herbs are used instead of isolated active ingredients (buffering). Although two samples of a particular herbal drug may contain constituent compounds in different proportions, practitioners claim that this does not generally cause clinical problems. There is some experimental evidence for synergy and buffering in certain whole-plant preparations,[176] but how far this can be generalized to all herbal products is not known.

2. *Herb combining.* Often, several different herbs are used together. Practitioners may say that the principles of synergy and buffering apply to combinations of plants and claim that combining herbs improves efficacy and reduces adverse effects.[‡] This contrasts with conventional practice, where polypharmacy is generally avoided to the extent possible, at least insofar as concurrent use of multiple preparations for the same purpose goes.

3. *Diagnosis.* Herbal practitioners may use different diagnostic principles from those used by conventional practitioners. For example, when treating arthritis, they might observe "underfunctioning of a patient's systems of elimination" and decide that the arthritis results from "an accumulation of metabolic waste products." A diuretic, choleretic, or laxative combination of herbs might then be prescribed alongside herbs with anti-inflammatory properties.

Safety

The history of herbal medicine use in general suggests a lack of efficacy. However, the long history of such use should not also be taken as an indication that those medications have been safe. While it is probably reasonable, as a rule, to assume that an herb that enjoyed wide use for a considerable period of time is not *acutely* toxic *when used in the traditional manner*, such assumptions leave open larger questions of chronic toxicities. Indeed, such products as comfrey (which is hepatotoxic and carcinogenic)[177,178] and tobacco were widely used for hundreds of years (in the case of tobacco, it was even endorsed by the medical profession). Concerns about long-term adverse effects might have been irrelevant in light of the short life spans of previous cultures—they are certainly not today. However, even had concerns about chronic toxicities been noted previously, they would likely have not been of great concern, as there was no real alternative to their use.

Although most herbal medicines are generally considered safe, herbal medicine probably presents a greater risk of adverse effects and interactions than

---

[‡]From A. Vickers, C. E. Zolman, ABC of complementary medicine: Herbal medicine. (*BMJ* 1999; 16[7216]: 1050–53). Example of an herbal prescription for osteoarthritis: Turmeric (*Curcuma longa*) tincture 20 ml (for anti-inflammatory activity and to "improve local circulation" at affected joints); Devil's claw (*Harpagophytum procumbens*) tincture 30 ml (for anti-inflammatory activity and general well-being); Ginseng (*Panax* spp.) tincture 10 ml (for weakness and exhaustion); White willow (*Salix alba*) tincture 20 ml (for anti-inflammatory activity); Liquorice (*Glycyrrhiza glabra*) 5 ml (for anti-inflammatory activity and to improve palatability and absorption of herbal medicine); Oats (*Avena sativa*) 15 ml (to aid sleep and for general well-being).

any other CAVM therapy. Allergic reactions, toxic reactions, adverse effects related to an herb's desired pharmacological actions, and possible mutagenic effects have been identified.[179] Reported adverse effects include germander with acute hepatitis, ephedra with fatal cardiovascular events, and comfrey with veno-occlusive disease.[180] Reports show that severe side effects and relevant interactions with other drugs can occur with herbal preparations. For example, hypericum extracts can decrease the concentration of a variety of other drugs by enzyme induction.[181] Several reviews summarizing side effects and interactions have been published.[182,183,184,185,186] In perhaps the most notorious instance in human medicine, rapidly progressive interstitial renal fibrosis and urothelial carcinoma have been reported in women taking Chinese herbs for weight reduction.[187]

Herbal products may also be contaminated, adulterated, or misidentified. In 1998, the California Department of Health reported that 32 percent of Asian patent medicines sold in that state contained undeclared pharmaceuticals or heavy metals;[188] this appears to be a particular problem in herbal preparations from Asian sources.[189,190,191] Similarly, PC-SPES was a patented "herbal" preparation designed for the treatment of human prostate problems, and positive reports even appeared in major medical journals. However, chemical analysis of the product revealed the presence of diethylstilbestrol, indomethacin, warfarin, or a combination of those drugs,[192] and it was subsequently removed from the marketplace (with criminal prosecution following). Because of such problems, calls for tighter regulation of botanical medicines have appeared.[193]

Veterinary Herbal and Botanical Medicine

The caveats and concerns regarding human applications of herbal and botanical veterinary medicines would be expected to be identical to those in human medicine.[194] Controlled studies on the clinical effects of herbal or botanical preparations in veterinary medicine appear to be absent. Doses are generally proportional to those used in human herbal medicine; however, it should be kept in mind that experience with pharmaceuticals has shown that extrapolating dosage or toxicity data from one species to another can be dangerous.

Due to their inherent toxicity, some herbal remedies should almost certainly not be used under any circumstance. Others, such as tea tree oil, while safe at some dilutions, can cause significant adverse effects.[195] In addition, because some herbal remedies contain multiple, biologically active constituents, interaction with conventional drugs is also a concern.[196] There is a newly formed Veterinary Botanical Medicine Association that appears to be attempting to promote the use of herbal remedies in animals.[197]

ELECTRICITY AND MAGNETISM

Historical

Throughout history, as today, medical acceptance of electricity and magnetism for routine therapy has been limited by the inability to confirm significant physiological effects from the employed fields.§ Benjamin Franklin, in the Paris of the 1780s, found physiological effects of static magnets impossible to isolate. Later, a research article in the 1892 *New York Medical Journal* reported on a series of studies performed in Thomas Edison's New Jersey laboratory to establish what, if any, physiological effect electromagnetic fields might possess. The investigations consisted of placing various samples of tissue, as well as living frogs, dogs, and people, between the poles of electromagnets that could produce magnetic fields with strengths more than twenty-five thousand times those of the earth's 0.55 gauss (55,000 nT) field. The authors reviewed each of their experiments and found that even intense electromagnetic field exposure did not alter physiological function in any of their circulatory, cellular, neurological, or respiratory studies. The authors concluded that they were unable to establish either the existence of effects or a physiological basis for electromagnetic therapy.[198] Today, in spite of numerous theories about how magnetic fields *might* cause physiological effects,[199] no theories have been confirmed. Indeed, people are routinely placed in fields much stronger than those used in therapy during MRI examinations without detectable detriment or changes in function. In addition, the mechanisms proposed to explain the putative effects of magnetic therapy generally do not seem plausible when extended to biological systems.

Static Magnetic Fields

Magnetic devices that radiate an unchanging magnetic field are available in a variety of configurations such as pads, bandages, blankets, and mattresses (for pets, too). A mechanism of action by which such devices might exert these effects remains elusive. Hypotheses for an effect of a static field include influencing the electronic spin rate states of chemical reaction intermediates[200,201] and influencing cyclical changes in the physical state(s) of water.[202] Importantly, none of the proposed effects has been demonstrated in biological systems under physiological condition.[203] Indeed, a weak magnetic field has

---

Some material in "Electricity and Magnetism" is from D. W. Ramey, Magnetic and electromagnetic therapy (*Sci Rev Alt Med* 1998; 2[1]:13–19. Reprinted with permission, Prometheus Books, Amherst, NY).

§Electricity and magnetism certainly do have legitimate uses in medicine, for example, in diagnostic magnetic resonance imaging, transcranial electromagnetic stimulation, or electroconvulsive therapy for psychotic major depression.

scarcely any effects on various biological functions of cells,[204] and it is difficult to understand how they might have effects in larger organisms.

Magnetic Pad Design

Manufacturers of magnetic pads may assert that alternating north and south magnetic poles can increase their putative effects. Alternating magnetic poles are most commonly seen in refrigerator magnets. By alternating the magnetic poles, an increased magnetic gradient is created, which increases the ability of the magnets to stick to the refrigerator. However, this increased strength is limited to a very short range; alternating fields tend to cancel each other out as they extend from the magnet. Also, there does not appear to be any consensus in the industry as to the ideal design for the pads. In fact, since tissues are three dimensional, there can be no preferred arrangement of the magnetic field applied. Whatever the design, magnets cannot work if there is no magnetic field applied, and at least one study has shown that the magnetic field strength of commercially available magnetic pads may be significantly lower than advertised.[205]

Still other mechanistic claims may be made for the "negative" pole of the magnet. These are quite clearly bogus. While magnets may indeed by marked with "+" and "−" signs, this indicates a relation to the electrical field. Magnets do not have negative poles.

Pulsating Electromagnetic Field Therapy (PEMF)

Michael Faraday discovered that an electric current passing through a wire coil could generate a magnetic field. Conversely, a changing magnetic field can generate an electric voltage; the magnetic field must change to have any electrical effect. The varying magnetic field from such devices rises and falls rhythmically in a pulse; hence, the term *pulsating electromagnetic field therapy* (PEMF), which generates rising and falling levels of a magnetic field and may induce electric current in tissue.

Mechanical and electrical stimuli help regulate extracellular matrix synthesis and repair, although the precise nature of such electromechanical signals is not known. In bone, signaling pathways may occur in cell membrane.[206,207] In soft tissue, alternating current electrical fields induce a redistribution of integral cell membrane proteins, which hypothetically could initiate signal transduction cascades and cause a reorganization of cytoskeletal structures.[208] However, the hypothesis that electrical signals may be responsible for information transfer in or to cells has been neither proved nor disproved.

There is ample evidence that electrical activity exists in the body at all times. For example, electrical currents can be measured in the beating heart and are also generated in the production of bone.[209] Thus, it is theorized that application of an appropriate electrical current, either directly through wires or indirectly through induction by a magnetic field, may affect tissues in several ways. The word *appropriate* is important since cells and tissues respond to a variety of electrical signal configurations in ways that suggest a degree of specificity for both the tissue affected and the signal itself. So far, attempts at determining the boundaries of such specificity has been unrewarding.

Clinical Studies on Magnetic Fields and Blood Flow

Proponents of applying static magnetic field therapy to injured or painful tissues may attribute therapeutic effects to an increase in local blood circulation. Unfortunately, the preponderance of scientific evidence does not support this hypothesis. First of all, the goal of increasing local blood circulation is perhaps illusory; the body controls the circulation of blood rather precisely, and there is only so much blood to go around. Nevertheless, a number of studies have investigated the effects of static magnetic fields on blood flow, and virtually every one of them has failed to demonstrate an effect. There are several reasons for this.

First of all, the theory is implausible. Although blood, like all tissues, contains electrically charged ions, and magnetic fields do exert a force on a moving ionic current (Faraday's law), two facts account for the lack of effect. First, the magnetic field applied to the tissue is extremely weak. Second, the flow of the ionic current (i.e., the blood) is extremely slow. Furthermore, any magnetic forces generated by a static field affecting fluid movement in blood vessels would have to overcome both the normal, pressure-driven turbulent flow of blood and the normal thermal-induced Brownian movement of the particles suspended in the blood. Given the strong physical forces that already exist in a blood vessel, any physical forces generated by a static magnetic field on flowing blood, particularly those as weak as the ones associated with therapeutic magnetic pads, are extremely unlikely to have a biological effect.

Numerous studies have confirmed this unlikelihood. No effect of dental magnets on the circulation of blood in the cheek could be demonstrated.[210] Scintigraphic evaluation of blood flow in mice exposed to two strengths of pulsating electromagnetic field force failed to demonstrate any circulatory effects.[211] A study on the circulatory effects of a magnetic foil was unable to show any effect in the skin of human forearms[212] or hands.[213] One study of horses showed that application of a magnetic pad over the tendon region for 24 hours showed no evidence of temperature increase in treated limbs versus placebo controlled limbs, using thermographic measurements as an indirect assessment of blood circulation to the area,[214] and direct measurements using quantitative scintigraphy, comparing a magnetized and a demagnetized pad, also failed to show an effect.[215]

As a more practical matter, if a magnet caused local increases in circulation, one would expect the area under the magnet to feel warm or become red as a result. Such an effect is not reported when magnets are held in the human hand. Furthermore, one would expect any circulatory effects produced by very weak magnetic fields to be magnified in stronger magnetic fields. However, no circulatory effects have ever been reported in magnetic resonance imaging machines, in which the magnetic forces generated are two to four orders of magnitude greater than those produced by therapeutic magnetic pads. In studies of humans exposed to magnetic fields up to 1 tesla (10,000 gauss), there was no evidence of alterations in local blood flow at the skin of the thumb or at the forearm.[216] Even extremely strong fields of 10 tesla are predicted to change the vascular pressure in a model of human vasculature by less than 0.2 percent, and experimental results of the effects of strong magnetic fields on concentrated saline solutions are in general agreement with these predictions.[217]

Based on the available scientific data, one must conclude that if there is an effect of magnetic fields on blood circulation, there is no known biological mechanism by which that effect is generated and that such effects cannot be reliably demonstrated experimentally. One may also postulate that the boots, blankets, and bandages in which the magnets are sewn have some sort of a thermal effect that is independent of the magnetic field (and could be duplicated with any form of bandaging).

Pulsating Electromagnetic Fields and Fractures

The most widely studied application of electromagnetic field therapy in human medicine is in fracture therapy. Although the mechanisms remain undetermined, several studies report that electrical fields generated by pulsating electromagnetic field therapy stimulate biologic processes pertinent to osteogenesis[218,219,220] and bone graft incorporation.[221,222] This form of therapy is approved for the treatment of delayed and nonunion fractures in humans in the United States by the United States Food and Drug Administration, and the effectiveness of the treatment is supported by small double-blind studies.[223] However, pulsating electromagnetic field therapy delayed the healing of fresh experimentally induced fractures in rabbits[224] and did not appear to assist the healing of fresh fractures in rats.[225] Other studies have failed to identify any beneficial effect of applying a magnetic field to a nonhealing fracture and concluded that the long periods of immobilization and inactivity required for the application of the magnetic field therapy were just as likely to be responsible for tissue healing as the application of the electromagnetic device.[226] Of course, the time of application and inactivity required for the use of such devices may limit their utility in veterinary medicine.

Magnetic Fields and Soft Tissues

Pulsating electromagnetic field therapy (PEMF) has been evaluated in the treatment of soft tissue injuries, with the results of some studies providing evidence that this form of therapy may be of value in promoting healing of chronic wounds (such as bedsores),[227] in neuronal regeneration,[228,229] and in many other soft tissue injuries.[230,231] Results of a study in an experimental Achilles tendinitis model in rats indicated that there was an initial decrease in water content in injured tendons treated with pulsating electromagnetic field therapy but that all treated groups were equal to controls by 14 days.[232] However, PEMF caused a decrease in tensile strength and an increase in peritendinous adhesions in a chicken flexor tendon model.[233] Purported effects (positive or negative) of PEMF in the treatment of tendon injuries are difficult to understand, as there appears to be a lack of significant electrical activity in tendons that could be altered by a pulsating electromagnetic field.

Criticisms of pulsating electromagnetic field studies include: some of the studies are poorly designed; independent trials have not been conducted to confirm positive results; and the electrical fields induced by the machines are several orders of magnitude lower than are required to alter the naturally occurring electrical fields that exist across biological membranes.[234] Much work needs to be done to optimize such variables as signal configuration and duration of treatment before pulsating electromagnetic field therapy can be generally recommended.

Magnetic Fields and Pain Relief

Both static and pulsating electromagnetic field therapy have also been promoted as being beneficial for the relief of pain. Objective clinical support for such applications is tenuous and conflicting. Thus, while one study may find magnetic fields beneficial in a specific condition, others, as well or better done, will find no effect in another.

As with other proposed effects, there is no known mechanism of action by which application of a magnetic field reduces pain. However, if they are effective in the relief of pain, it is unlikely that the effect is related to a reduction in nerve conductivity; the field required to produce a 10 percent reduction in nerve conductivity is roughly 24 tesla,[235] a field of a strength that can only be created in the laboratory. High-intensity magnetic field pulses can depolarize superficial and deep nerves, creating a 30–40 minute antinociceptive effect to both mechanical and heat stimuli in rats, but the clinical relevance of such an effect is not known.[236]

Studies evaluating the effects of pulsating electromagnetic fields in the relief of pain have shown conflicting results. Pulsating electromagnetic field therapy has reportedly provided pain relief in the treatment of osteoarthritis of the human knee and cervical spine,[237,238] in the treatment of persistent neck pain,[239] and in the treatment of women with chronic refractory pelvic pain.[240] However, electromagnetic therapy showed no benefit in the relief of pain due to shoulder arthritis,[241] and a 1994 summary of published trials of

nonmedicinal and noninvasive therapies for hip and knee osteoarthritis concluded that there were insufficient data available to draw any conclusions on
the efficacy of the therapy.[242] Paradoxically, another study in humans showed
that magnetic treatment actually induced hyperalgesia in a tooth pain model.[243]
Regardless, the evidence for such effects does not appear to be accumulating.

Pads that apply a static magnetic field are also promoted as having pain-
relieving effects. Early, poorly controlled studies from the Japanese literature
suggest that static magnetic devices were highly effective in alleviating subjective symptoms such as neck, shoulder, and other muscular pain.[244,245] One
controlled, double-blind pilot study suggested that magnetic pads were effective in the relief of myofascial or arthritislike pain in postpolio syndrome,[246]
although every patient in the study, whether being treated with a placebo or a
magnet, showed relief from pain. Other studies have suggested that static
magnets were useful in relieving the neuropathic foot pain associated with diabetes[247,248] or that static magnets reduced pain and enhanced functional movement in human patients with osteoarthritis of the knee.[249]

However, still other studies have concluded that a magnetic foil offered
no advantage over plain insoles in the treatment of pain of the human
heel,[250] that a magnetic necklace had no effect on neck and shoulder pain,[251]
and that magnetic insoles had no effect on human heel pain.[252] In addition,
magnetic pads had no effect on back pain,[253] a finding that confirmed a large
consumer survey in which magnets helped back pain "only a little or not at
all" in 50 percent or more cases.[254] It has also been suggested that there is a
strong placebo effect at work in the perception of pain relief offered by static magnetic devices.[255] Such effects may also be seen in animal owners, who
may see effects of treatment on their animals when, in fact, no improvement
occurs.

Magnetic Fields in Veterinary Medicine

While applications of pulsating electromagnetic fields in small animals appear
to be infrequent, devices may be applied to horses with boots or blankets.
Some of the variables of the magnetic field generated (such as the amplitude
and frequency of the signal) can be controlled using this form of magnetic
therapy. However, changes in these variables appear to affect different tissues
in different ways, and those ways are not well defined, making selection of
ideal field strength of the therapy problematic.

Static magnetic devices are widely advertised in magazines targeted at animal owners, and products such as magnetic pet mattresses and equine leg
wraps, blankets, and hoof pads are available. These products produce an
extremely low static magnetic influence on the targeted tissue; the magnetic
field cannot be modulated or, in some cases, even measured. The principal
advantage of this form of magnetic therapy is that it is relatively inexpensive

(compared to the cost of the machines) and easy to apply. The disadvantage is that as yet there is no scientific evidence of a physiological effect.

There are no published scientific studies available that demonstrate that any form of magnetic field therapy is valuable in the treatment of disease conditions of animals. Daily electromagnetic therapy appeared to increase the concentration of blood vessels in surgically created defects of equine superficial digital flexor tendon, but the maturation of the repair tissue and the transformation of collagen type (two essential components in the healing process of tendon) actually were delayed by the treatment in tendon samples collected at 8 to 12 weeks after surgery.[256] No benefit could be demonstrated in the healing of freshly created bone injuries treated with pulsating electromagnetic field therapy when compared to untreated control limbs,[257] although another study did suggest an increase in bone activity under pulsating electromagnetic field treatment when holes were drilled in horse cannon bones.[258] Topical treatment with a pulsed electromagnetic field showed little effect on metabolism of normal horse bone in another study.[259]

Safety

Concerns about the safety of electrical, magnetic, and electromagnetic field exposure seem to have arisen in the last 30 years. In addition, the role of the "electromagnetic underdog," the brave outsider who is willing to challenge the hoary skeptics, has changed from that of attacking the establishment for resisting the acceptance (due to alleged selfish and self-seeking reasons) of a valuable new treatment, to that of attacking the establishment for hiding the detrimental effects of these fields (again, due to alleged selfish and self-seeking reasons).

More specifically, safety issues seem to have come to the forefront in the late 1970s and early 1980s with a series of epidemiological studies that often appeared to establish a link between occupational exposure to electromagnetic fields and an increased incidence of leukemia.[260] These occupational surveys were supplemented by additional epidemiological investigations of the household exposure of children and adults to ambient electromagnetic fields, surveys that frequently found increased incidences of breast cancer, abnormal pregnancies, chromosomal aberrations, and congenital deformities in association with increased electromagnetic field exposure.[261]

While these associations are a concern, a number of caveats are appropriate. For example, many analyses find no links. In addition, the early studies that found associations were pioneer efforts that, with hindsight, inaccurately estimated EMF exposures and neglected confounding factors such as exposure to chemical toxins. In all, mixed findings, faulty exposure estimates, incomplete recognition of confounding variables, questionable assumptions, and extensive statistical manipulation limit the robustness of any association between EMF exposure and detrimental health effects.[262] At this point, it seems best to follow the lead of a recent National Research Council panel, which, after noting that early epidemiological studies suggested an association between low-intensity EMF fields and increased rates of cancer, stated that more recent and better-designed studies support the view that there is "no conclusive and consistent evidence" that EMF exposure causes significant increases in the risks of cancer or neurobehavioral or reproductive dysfunction.[263]

ELECTRICITY

Various applications of electricity have found use in medicine today. For example, in human physical therapy, higher intensity electrical stimulation is used to help muscles regain strength and to elicit movement and improve function in paralyzed limbs. The United States Food and Drug Administration has approved lower intensity devices for use in assisting in fracture healing. In other applications, such as wound healing or pain management, the use of electricity is still investigational.

Transcutaneous electrical nerve stimulation (TENS) devices have gained some acceptance in the treatment of human pain of various origins, however, the mechanism of action remains unclear. The units consist of a battery, an electrical signal generator, and a set of electrodes and are capable of generating a variety of electrical stimuli of differing currents and pulses, although the clinical relevance of the various choices is unclear. Electrodes are typically placed over the painful area, although numerous other sites may be chosen, including putative acupuncture points.

Acceptance of and long-term success for electrical therapies has been elusive. Good clinical support is mixed; some conditions may be more amenable to them than others. Thus, while analyses may find that TENS therapy is useful for the treatment of osteoarthritis of the human knee,[264] it has not been shown to be effective for acute or chronic low back pain in people.[265]

Other applications of electricity may also report effectiveness for certain conditions. In particular, electricity is sometimes applied at acupuncture points, either via inserted needles or noninvasive pads (both may be referred to as electroacupuncture).[266] Although there is occasional evidence of efficacy, such interventions blur the distinction between electricity and acupuncture, call into question the existence of acupuncture points,[267] and certainly call into question whether needle penetration is necessary to achieve an effect of the applied electricity.

Safety

Electrical therapy presents few issues regarding safety. In humans, contact dermatitis and skin irritation may be reported.[268] Of course, intense applications of electricity can be uncomfortable, but this is easily corrected when settings are changed. In humans, application of electrical devices to pregnant women is generally avoided, although this is because of an abundance of caution, rather than because of supporting clinical data.

ENERGY MEDICINE

Many people mistakenly believe that the universe is composed primarily of two kinds of things.

1. Matter, which includes the bodies of living organisms and the other material of the universe. They may have heard that matter is composed of particulate atoms, and may associate material objects with notions of discreteness and scientific reductionism.
2. Energy, which is sometimes associated—especially in the scientifically naïve mind—with spirit or soul.

The common belief is that living things possess some special quality that makes them alive, that is, a vital force of living energy. Some alternative theorists may associate this energy with physical electromagnetic fields (which, to be fair, do appear to be somewhat mysterious to many people, even more than a century after their discovery). In general, these energy fields seem to be associated with notions of continuity and holism, notions that are said to oppose the discreteness and reductionism of cold science and modern medicine.

Reductionism attempts to explain complex sets of facts, entities, phenomena, or structures by simpler sets. Science has advanced by reductionism. Indeed, science's understanding of the world has come by examining smaller and smaller pieces of it. When those pieces are assembled, they help explain the whole. On the other hand, bioenergetics is offered as a "holistic" approach, treating the "whole" animal. In this sense, holistic does not refer to the importance of recognizing that many factors, including the psychological, emotional, and social, may contribute to an organism's overall sense of well-being. However, treating the whole animal does not contradict any of the principles of reductionism, nor does the fact that parts of physical systems interact with one another.

In modern permutations, the vital force may be referred to as the *bioenergetic field*. However, the use of the term *bioenergetic* is somewhat ambiguous. In its conventional use, the term refers to exchanges of energy within organisms, as well as those between those organisms and their environment. These occur by normal chemical and physical processes that can be readily measured. However, this is apparently not what modern vitalists have in mind. Instead, they imagine the bioenergetic field as a ubiquitous force that pervades the universe.

"Energy Medicine" was writtten with Victor Stenger, PhD.

The exact nature of the proposed bioenergetic field remains elusive, although proponents thereof may give clues to its existence. For example, one veterinary author identifies the bioenergetic field with the classic electromagnetic field, while at the same time confusing it with quantum fields or wave functions. She asserts that, "the principles of energy medicine originate in quantum physics. Bioenergetic medicine is the study of human and animal bodies as dynamic electromagnetic fields existing in an electromagnetic environment. . . . Based on Einstein's theories of quantum physics,** these energetic concepts are being integrated into medicine for a comprehensive approach to disease diagnosis, prevention and treatment."[269]

However, beliefs in vital energies do not reflect the developments that have occurred in either the physical or biological sciences of the past several centuries. In the late nineteenth century, most scientists (as most scientifically naïve people today) held that energy and matter were separate and distinct substances. Matter, while appearing continuous to the naked eye, was known to be composed of discrete, localized atoms. Light had been shown to be a form of an electromagnetic wave, which was believed to result from the vibration of a continuous cosmic field, the aether. Electromagnetic waves were thought to be a form of pure energy. Gravity was thought to be a continuous action-at-a-distance field.

In the twentieth century, these views evolved and changed. Energy and matter were recognized to be equivalent, as signified by Einstein's famous equation $E = mc^2$. The discrete nature of matter was fully confirmed. Energy was shown to occur, like matter, in discrete lumps called *quanta* (this was Max Planck's discovery that triggered the development of quantum mechanics). Light was found to be composed of particulate matter called *photons*. The theory of general relativity explains gravity in terms of the curvature of space rather than as a continuous force field. No evidence has been found for any continuous medium in the universe.

The fact remains that no unique living force has ever been conclusively demonstrated to exist in scientific experiments. Of course, it is still *possible* that a life force might someday be found, but this is not what is claimed in the literature that promotes much of CAVM. It would seem that the effects of these mysterious forces in living things would be easily detectable, given the great precision with which physical phenomena can be measured. For example, physics can measure the magnetic dipole moment of the electron (a measure of the

---

** While Einstein certainly contributed to the development of quantum mechanics, especially with photon theory, modern quantum physics is the result of a large group of physicists, including Planck, Bohr, de Broglie, Heisenberg, among many others. Einstein's fame rests securely enough on his two theories of relativity. Einstein actually objected to quantum mechanics, saying famously, "God does not play dice."

strength of the electron's magnetic field) to one part in ten billion, and calculate it with the same accuracy. It surely should be able to detect forces in the body that are capable of moving atoms around or somehow physically altering the course of disease. But neither physics nor any other science has seen anything that suggests that such forces exist. Alternative concepts of bioenergetics directly contradict known physical laws, and, as such, are nonscientific.

The Standard Model of Matter

Material objects are made up of atoms, which in turn are composed of nuclei and electrons. Nuclei are composed of protons and neutrons, which them-selves are composed of quarks. By the 1970s, the picture of matter and energy had been strongly established in what is still called the *standard model*, but is now a fully developed and highly successful theory. Under this model, the fun-damental constituents of matter could logically be grouped into families of subatomic particles.

The Standard Model of Forces

The elementary particles that make up matter are only half of the story. The standard model also tells how these particles interact with one another to make up the more complex matter that has evolved into stars, planets, and animals. In the standard model, forces result from the exchange of particles.

Quantum fields in quantum theory describe these force particles. No con-tinuous medium, special energy, or vital force is involved.

Quantum Fields

Quantum fields are strictly theoretical objects, like the density field that describes the average behavior of particulate matter. They do not describe a continuous energy that pervades space. Since every particle is the quantum of a quantum field, no fields exist independently from other particles. Further-more, quanta do not act instantaneously over space. Their effects propagate no faster than the speed of light.

According to energy medicine proponents, quantum mechanics is said to provide a basis for a mind-matter connection. This notion appears to arise from the fact that, in quantum mechanics, the act of observation interferes with what is being observed, as expressed by the *Heisenberg uncertainty princi-ple*. In 1927, Werner Heisenberg theorized that the position and momentum of a particle could not be simultaneously measured with high precision. Howev-er, Heisenberg's principle is not a statement about the inaccuracy of measure-ment instruments, nor is it a reflection on the quality of experimental meth-ods; it arises from the wave properties inherent in the quantum mechanical description of nature. Even with perfect instruments and technique, the uncertainty is inherent in the nature of things.

However, the uncertainty principle is sometimes perverted to suggest that reality is determined by consciousness; that it's not possible to be certain of anything; otherwise stated, that one makes one's own reality. Such an interpretation is quite simply wrong. There is no such implication inherent in the Heisenberg principle, nor in quantum phenomena or quantum theory.

No evidence for any special vital forces, energies, auras, or fields has ever been found in modern science. Modern physics has shown that energy and matter are the same entity and finds no evidence for continuous fields. The quantum fields of theoretical physics are directly connected, one to one, to particles, the quanta of the fields. A consistent picture of elementary particles and forces that successfully describes all current observations exists within the framework of the standard model. Living matter is composed of the same particles acted on by the same forces as nonliving matter. Quantum mechanics provides no basis for paranormal or holistic claims (in spite of the unbridled use of the word *quantum*), while all of modern physics remains totally materialistic and reductionistic.

LASER AND LIGHT THERAPY

Various colored light devices may be sold as diagnostic or therapeutic, most consisting of arrays of inexpensive red-light-emitting diodes (LEDs), diode lasers such as those used in laser pointers, or even flashlights with colored tips. Such devices are uniformly without therapeutic value and have no scientific base of support. If they caused enough heat, there could be some thermal effect; however, this is not what proponents of such therapies claim.

For light devices to be therapeutic, a chromophore molecule in the body must first absorb their light, which causes the molecule to briefly reach a higher energy level (photoexcitation). Then, a therapeutically useful photochemical reaction must occur (the longer-energy wavelengths of visible light only affect chemical bonds and do not lead to photochemical reactions). Unfortunately, most molecules in the body have no color, do not absorb visible light, and do not undergo photoexcitation; thus, the typical light therapy using visible light is essentially worthless. With the exception of the photoactive pigments in the eye, the main compounds that do absorb visible light are melanin, the pigment of skin, and heme-containing proteins, such as exist in the blood. However, these compounds do not undergo photochemical reactions in vivo; they are metabolically inert. Thus, it is not surprising that light

---

Some material in "Laser and Light Therapy" is adapted from D. W. Ramey and J. R. Basford, A review of laser therapy in the horse (*Compendium on Continuing Education*, March 2000. Reprinted with permission, Veterinary Learning Systems, Yardley, PA).

therapy using visible light—no matter what color—rarely seems to have a beneficial physiological effect.[270]

Laser (light amplification by stimulated emission of radiation) light has three important characteristics that distinguish it from other forms of light: coherency (i.e., the light waves are in phase), collimation (i.e., the light beam is narrow), and monochromaticity (i.e., pure color). Not all of these characteristics seem important from a therapeutic standpoint, however. Coherency and collimation do not seem to be crucial as both rapidly degrade as the beam passes through tissue. Monochromaticity, however, appears to be essential as effects that occur at one wavelength are absent at another.[271]

Any number of low-intensity lasers have been used to treat humans and animals. The earliest studies used the visible 632.8 nm helium neon (HeNe) and ruby lasers. With time, infrared semiconductor lasers (wavelengths between 820 nm and 904 nm), such as the Gallium Arsenide (GaAs) and Gallium Aluminum Arsenide (GaAlAs), have become those most widely used.[272] HeNe devices are still widely used, especially in wound healing and treatment of various equine injuries. Most current treatments involve devices with output powers between 30 and 100 mW. However, in human medicine, as laser powers have increased, treatment times have tended to decrease. Thus, treatment dosages often remain at or near the levels established by the early investigators (1–4 J/cm^2).

Biophysics of Light Therapy

For light to be effective in treating tissues below the skin surface, obviously, the light must be able to reach those tissues. Light that is not absorbed by water, or by pigments such as hemoglobin and melanin, is attenuated in a gradual manner as it passes through tissue. This attenuation is best described as an exponential decrease produced by the scattering and absorption that occur as light passes through tissue. For example, the visible red light (632.8 nm) of a HeNe laser penetrates 0.5–1 mm before losing about a third (more precisely, 1/e, where e is the base of natural logarithm, approximately 2.718) of its intensity. Longer wavelengths are more resistant to scattering than are shorter ones.[273]

In vitro research suggests that even exposures of less than 0.01 Joules/cm^2 can alter cellular processes. Since laser therapy treatments typically involve the delivery of 1–4 + J/cm^2 to the skin, this means that laser beams can typically penetrate six to seven "penetration depths" before they are attenuated to levels that would be considered ineffective. This implies that laser beams can penetrate to a tissue depth of 0.5–2.5 cm in human tissues, with longer wavelengths penetrating more effectively. Thus, it seems reasonable to surmise that at least superficial nerves and tissues *might* respond to laser treatment in humans.

Far less is known about light penetration through animal skin. However, given that animals' skin is often considerably thicker than human skin and that it is covered with hair, it is reasonable to surmise that the subcutaneous penetration of light devices in animals may be considerably less than in humans.

Laboratory Research

The strongest support for laser therapy comes from in vitro research. Although some controversy persists, it seems well established that laser irradiation alters cellular processes in a nondestructive manner that is wavelength dependent but does not involve heating. Laser therapy involves such low powers that irradiation is imperceptible and produces temperature elevations of less than or equal to 0.5–0.75°C.[274,275]

Cellular processes, such as protein synthesis,[276] cell growth and differentiation,[277] and motility,[278] appear to be both stimulated and inhibited by laser irradiation. Alterations in cell binding affinities and energy production,[279] neurotransmitter release,[280] and phagocytosis[281] are also reported. The role of light in these processes is obscure and its mechanism of action is poorly understood, although it seems most likely that the resonant absorption of photons by respiratory chain components (in particular, cytochrome C) is important. However, explanations that lasers "increase blood flow," "reestablish the lymphatic system," or "stimulate endorphins" are simplistic, incomplete, and only sporadically supported by high-quality research.

The clinical value of low-intensity laser irradiation in the treatment of animals and humans is far less established. Early anecdotal clinical reports tended to be extremely favorable. Although research quality is improving, results remain controversial and difficult to evaluate.

Clinical Research—Human

Laser therapy has been advocated in the treatment of a broad array of human soft tissue, neurological, and inflammatory conditions. However, laser therapy has yet to show unequivocal effectiveness in the treatment of any human condition. There are tantalizing indications of benefits, but strong evidence of clear clinical benefits does not exist. Even in situations where benefits seem more probable, the optimal wavelengths, intensities, and dosages remain unknown. Furthermore, differing lasers, techniques, variable research quality, semiquantitative outcome measures (e.g., pain), and conflicting results make systematic evaluation of laser therapy difficult.

Laser therapy gained its first prominence in the treatment of human wounds. Poorly controlled reports in the late 1960s and early 1970s concluded that laser irradiation could heal equal to or greater than 70 percent of human lower extremity ulcers that had been refractory to other treatment.[282] As a result, while they focused attention on laser therapy, they have had a limited role in gaining laser therapy acceptance into mainstream medicine. In contrast, the results of controlled and blinded studies indicate that neither HeNe[283,284] nor GaAs[285] laser irradiation is more effective than placebo treatments. Numerous data obtained from cell studies and animal experiments were reviewed in 2002. These studies failed to demonstrate unequivocal evidence to support the decision to conduct trials with low-level laser therapy and concluded that this type of phototherapy should not be considered a valuable adjuvant treatment for wound healing in humans.[286]

Tendon injuries and inflammation are among the most widely investigated laser therapy applications. Shoulder tendinitis was an early indication for laser therapy in humans. Unfortunately, initial clinical trials were generally open and uncontrolled, and they included a variety of diagnoses. Thus, while one study found patients with shoulder tendinitis benefiting from treatment,[287] another found no benefit.[288] Investigations of laser treatment of tendinopathies have failed to distinguish between laser and placebo treatments,[289] and there is evidence of no difference when laser therapy is compared with no treatment for therapy of acute or chronic Achilles tendinitis in humans.[290]

Early investigations found a decrease in pain, swelling, medication use, and morning stiffness after laser treatment in human rheumatoid arthritis,[291] a condition that, due to the superficial nature of joints, should be amenable to laser therapy. However, later, controlled studies often found no effect from laser therapy of rheumatoid arthritis,[292] and a single report exists in which clinical and laboratory signs of rheumatoid arthritis were worsened by low-intensity laser therapy.[293] Interest has subsequently fluctuated.

The response of human patients with osteoarthritis to laser therapy also has been mixed. Improvement in function and in pain relief of degenerative arthritis of the temporomandibular joint[294] and the knee[295] are reported, however, controlled and blinded studies fail to show beneficial effects in the treatment of osteoarthritis of the knee,[296] the thumb,[297] and acute sprains of the ankle.[298] As is true in so many areas, the mixture of lasers, powers, and study designs make evaluation difficult, as noted in a 2000 meta-analysis that concluded that data were lacking on appropriate wavelengths, treatment durations, dosages, and sites of application (e.g., over nerves instead of joints).[299]

In humans, pain relief, whether in the form of simple analgesia or in treatment of an underlying painful condition, is perhaps the most common indication for laser therapy. As is true with most clinical applications in humans, initial reports were extremely positive, but benefits became more subtle and difficult to establish as investigations became more rigorous.[300] One controlled study shows that tooth sensitivity is reduced after laser irradiation;[301] however, other such studies find that treatment may not lessen back,[302] lateral epicondylitis (tennis elbow),[303] ischemic,[304] or oral pain.[305] Trigger points (points that produce a well-described pattern of referred pain when pressed), a controversial but prominent feature of chronic pain, are reported to both benefit from[306] and not respond to low-level laser therapy.[307]

Professional Attitudes

Two surveys of professionals who may employ laser therapy have been reported. In the treatment of wounds, a 1992 survey of more than five hundred Dutch health professionals—dermatologists, as well as physicians and nurses working in nursing homes—were asked to rank treatments for pressure sores on a scale from 0 (harmful) to 10 (excellent). Pressure relief and patient education were ranked highly at 6.2–8.3. High-protein diets, hydrocolloid dressings, and zinc oxide were ranked intermediately (5.0–5.6). Laser therapy scored far lower at 1.5–3.1.[308]

As to its efficacy in pain relief, a 1994 survey of two hundred specialists in human rehabilitative medicine and rheumatology found fewer than 20 percent who believed that laser therapy was an effective modality in the treatment of musculoskeletal disease.[309] Conditions that were treated with laser therapy included acute arthritis, tendinitis, neck and back pain, and joint contracture.

In 2000, the Dutch Health Council published a report on the efficacy of electrotherapy, laser therapy, and ultrasound treatment for musculoskeletal disorders based on three systematic reviews, including 169 randomized clinical trials. The council found virtually no conclusive clinically relevant effects of the three forms of physical therapy, and called for further research before implementing such modalities in practice. Furthermore, they "strongly recommended" that the widespread use of electrotherapy, laser therapy, and ultrasound treatment should be reduced.[310]

Reviews and Meta-Analysis

A meta-analysis of 36 randomized laser therapy studies of musculoskeletal pain and skin disorders (such as chronic ulcers) was unable to draw any conclusions about the treatment of skin disorders and suggested that better investigations of musculoskeletal disorders showed a tendency for treatment to be more effective than placebo.[311] Despite the fact that more than 1,700 subjects were included in this study, variability of study design and quality limited the analysis and the investigators could find no clear relationship between the laser dosage applied and the efficacy of therapy.

A more strenuously restricted meta-analysis limited to 23 musculoskeletal pain trials found no differences between laser and placebo treatment in the studies that were deemed "adequately blinded" and less than a 10 percent difference in the "insufficiently blinded" subset. The authors concluded that low-level laser therapy has no proven effectiveness in the treatment of musculoskeletal pain.[312] A review of placebo-controlled, double-blind trials concluded that there is no particular disease or symptom that seems to uniquely respond to the therapy and suggests that laser therapy is neither clinically effective nor scientifically proven.[313] Other reviews have concluded that for the treatment of hip and knee osteoarthritis, more data were needed before laser therapy could be recommended.[314] A review of conservative management of mechanical neck disorders concluded that laser therapy was ineffective and recommended against its use.[315] Finally, a report by the Australian Health Technology Advisory Committee on low-power lasers in medicine observed that there is no agreed-upon theory to explain the mechanism of the proposed effects and no clear consensus on the optimal wavelengths, treatment approach, or conditions to be treated. The committee concluded that "the efficacy of low-power lasers in the treatment of musculoskeletal and other conditions is not established."[316]

Laser Acupuncture

As with other modalities, stimulation of putative acupuncture points with low-intensity lasers has been used at times in place of needle or acupressure techniques. Effectiveness has been difficult to establish. Uncontrolled reports typically find a large portion of the studied patients to be improved or cured after treatment. However, controlled studies of laser acupuncture tend to find it either without effect or less beneficial than traditional needle acupuncture.[317] Still other laser devices purport to automatically find acupuncture points (e.g., Centurion Systems, Edison, NJ), a remarkable claim indeed given the lack of proof for the existence of such points.

Clinical Research—Animals

Extrapolation to animals of benefits seen in humans treated with light therapy is made difficult by the fact that the conditions for which laser therapy is used in human medicine often do not have an exact counterpart in animals. Nevertheless, a number of animal applications of light therapy have been investigated.

Laboratory and animal studies offer mixed support for laser application to healing wounds. For example, some studies find that laser irradiation stimulates capillary growth, collagen deposition, granulation tissue formation, and fibroblast activity, and lessens inflammation.[318,319] Other studies have concluded that laser irradiation may either enhance, inhibit, or have no effect on the function of a variety of microorganisms and cells[320] and that there is no effect of HeNe radiation on a variety of cellular components of wound healing.[321]

Acceleration of wound healing following laser irradiation has been reported in diabetic mice with chronic wounds,[322] in experimentally induced full thickness teat wounds in dairy cattle,[323] and in rat wounds,[324,325] among others. However, studies in rabbits and rats find that while laser irradiation may speed repair in the early stages of wound healing, the effects may be clinically insignificant.[326,327,328] In fact, other studies report that laser irradiation has no effect on healing in a variety of animals, including at least six studies in rats[329] as well as guinea pigs,[330] swine,[331] and beagle dogs.[332] Finally, a randomized, controlled, and blinded study of second intention wound healing (open, unsutured wounds) in horses treated with a low-intensity GaAlAs laser showed no difference in wound contraction and epithelialization between laser-treated and control wounds and concluded that laser treatment had no significant effect.[333]

In the only histopathologic study of laser therapy in horses, surgical incisions were made in the skin and superficial digital flexor tendons in horses. The limbs were then treated with a low-intensity laser therapy device of unreported type. At the completion of treatment, skin and superficial digital flexor tendons from incised laser-irradiated, incised-control, and nonincised-control limbs were compared microscopically. The investigators, who were blinded, were unable to find qualitative differences between laser irradiated and nonirradiated tissues.[334]

Treatment of superficial tendon and ligament injuries appears to be one of the most commonly suggested uses of low-intensity laser therapy in horses. A noncontrolled, nonblinded report of 42 Standardbreds with "chronic bowed tendons," which were racing within 120 days of treatment with an infrared 904 nm laser, suggested dramatic improvement following laser therapy.[335] On the other hand, a retrospective study of factors affecting the clinical outcome of injuries to the superficial digital flexor tendon in a group of National Hunt racehorses in England found no statistically significant differences between horses treated with a laser of unreported type and intensity and untreated groups, although the results from laser-treated horses tended to be not as good as those horses treated conservatively.[336] Unfortunately, in neither of these studies are the lasers and dosages specified nor are the treatments controlled for the severity or duration of the injury.

Low-intensity laser irradiation appeared to be effective in promoting healing of experimentally induced equine pharyngeal ulcers in one unblinded study.[337] Three poorly defined and unrelated conditions (pharyngeal lymphoid hyperplasia, "check ligament injuries," and "chronic plantar desmitis") were treated in an another uncontrolled study with a 904 nm infrared laser.[338]

Low-level laser application to acupuncture points of the equine back has been described as being effective for the treatment of chronic back pain in 10 of 14 horses, in one uncontrolled and unblinded study based on clinical exam and performance level acceptable to the owner of the horse.[339] In a similar uncontrolled and unblinded study, laser application to acupuncture points was deemed as effective as needling or injection in horses with back pain of 2 to 108 months duration.[340] Of course, such investigations of back pain in horses are hampered by the lack of objective criteria on which to base a diagnosis, as well as by the lack of blinding and other methods used in an effort to ensure that trials are of high quality.

Laser or light devices for animals may be accompanied by a variety of claims that are poorly substantiated. For example, promotional literature for some light devices asserts that light therapy can be used as an effective treatment for many disease conditions of many animals (e.g., Equi-Light Therapy Systems, Odessa, FL, and its claims for the treatment of horses, elephants, black rhinos, penguins, whales, dogs, cats, snakes, and "more").[341]

Of course, clinical considerations are not the only ones useful in evaluating therapies. Given the difficulty in establishing clinical effects, the relatively modest effects demonstrated (when effects can be demonstrated) and the cost of such devices, one may reasonably conclude that the benefits from light therapy devices may not be worth the cost.

Safety

Devices that project visible light or varying colors provide such low power that harming the patient is virtually inconceivable. Furthermore, the powers used in laser therapy are, by definition, too low to damage or destroy tissue either by heating or nonlinear acoustic effects. Literature searches do not reveal a substantive risk from low-level laser therapy. Human patients may comment about transient warmth or tingling shortly after treatment, however, this often occurs in both laser- and placebo-treated subjects.[313]

Direct observation of a 1 mW HeNe (visible red light) beam can produce a headache even though beams of 5 mW neither stimulate nociceptors nor produce more than a 0.1°C temperature change in the cornea.[342] In any case, retinal damage is a concern and therapists and patients should use protective glasses and avoid looking directly at the beam or its reflection. Although there is no proven risk for low-intensity laser therapy, investigators in human medicine tend to avoid treating pregnant women, cancer patients, acute hemorrhages, growth plates, and photosensitive skin.[313]

8

Untested Therapies and Medical Anarchism

The privileged role in society assumed by practitioners of scientific medicine, human and animal, stems ultimately from society's desire for therapies and diagnoses based in empirical validation, with science being the method by which that empirical validation has been achieved. Serious criticisms of scientific medicine that merit serious attention have also been examined, some of which cast doubt on the suggestion that scientific medicine is as good as it could be. But however valid these criticisms discussed may be—and they may be significant enough to threaten the social foundations of biomedicine—they do not at all detract from the fundamental credo of scientific therapeutics and diagnostics, that is, that it is desirable to search for empirically verifiable, falsifiable, testable modalities. Even when scientific medicine deviates from its own ideal by utilizing unproven therapeutic modalities, as critics charge, that does not falsify the ideal of accepting only empirical evidence-based therapies, any more than the mathematician who makes a mistake on his taxes invalidates arithmetic.

As discussed earlier, but which bears repeating, for medical practitioners, enjoying special privileges in society, such as being allowed to perform surgery, write prescriptions, possess narcotics, and so on, logically rests upon their implicit commitment to scientifically validated, evidence-based, medicine. As long as society expects this of human and veterinary practitioners, and assumes adherence on the part of MDs and DVMs to a science-based approach when being granted professional status, it is in essence an ethical breach of contract to stray from empirically validated therapies except in the carefully circumscribed context of researching and testing new modalities, and there only when following the rules set for such professionals.

To do otherwise is to violate root principles of professional ethics in the most basic sense of the term. Professions, as has been mentioned, are granted special dispensations by society to fulfill some vital role. Furthermore, since the average member of society lacks the knowledge being a professional pre-supposes, society is loath to regulate professions in any detail. Thus, society essentially says to professions: you regulate yourselves the way we would regu-late you if we fully understood what you know and do (which we don't), and if you don't, we'll know about it and regulate you anyway. In veterinary medi-cine, this principle was well illustrated when Congress discovered that some veterinarians were cavalierly dispensing antibiotics to farms for promoting growth in animals, and thereby driving the evolution of antibiotic resistance. Congress's response was to propose legislation eliminating extra-label drug use for veterinarians, an action that would have made the practice of veteri-nary medicine exceedingly difficult, and that was narrowly averted.

The extra-label antibiotics case is significantly analogous to the situation with human and veterinary practitioners when they deviate from scientifically confirmed diagnostics and therapeutics. In the antibiotics case, veterinarians were bending to pressure from a certain constituency—farmers—at the expense of violating their presuppositional commitment to society in general not to endanger public health. By the same token, when MDs and DVMs bend to elements in society who demand nonscientifically based therapies and who are willing to spend upwards of $20 billion per year on such therapies, they do so at the expense of their implicit commitment to society to advance only sci-entific, evidentiary-based diagnostics and therapeutics. In addition, they may well violate the age-old fundamental ethical principle of all medicine to "do no harm."

With regard to that principle, veterinarians (and, in the human medical field, pediatricians) stand in a special position. While it is clearly wrong for a medical professional to dispense unproven therapeutic modalities in uncon-trolled situations without informed consent, one could argue that, in the case of a rational, competent adult patient, the patient is entitled to any therapy he or she chooses. However, this entitlement does not also mean that he or she must receive the therapy from a medical professional certified by society to be based in empirical science. It seems obvious that if a client prefers to have his or her animal(s) treated by some alternative to veterinary medicine, he or she should be able to choose to go to an alternative practitioner. But a child or ani-mal cannot choose, and, since the pediatrician's primary obligation is to the child, and the veterinarian's primary obligation is to the animal, he or she is bound morally to pursue only validated therapies, or to make sure that those therapies that *are* being employed are being evaluated so that they may be adopted or discarded, as the evidence leads. Indeed, society has defended the obligation of professionals to dispense, and the right of the patient to receive, proven therapies, as in the case of children who may receive a treatment even against parental wishes, such as when members of religious sects do not wish to have their children given life-saving transfusions, medicines, or surgeries.

The same is true for a veterinarian. As Plato said of a shepherd, the primary obligation of the shepherd, by the very nature of his role, is to the good of the sheep. His obligation to himself as wage earner is secondary to the imperative to care for the animals. Thus, no one would defend a shepherd who starved his sheep if bribed to do so or a veterinarian who broke a horse's leg to make more money for himself or for the client! Similarly, a veterinarian's role is to maintain health, alleviate suffering, or cure disease in animals, and to do so using validated therapies—the ones that are most likely to work—and not merely to employ untested or faddish modalities at the whim of the client. As professor of anesthesiology at the University of Illinois School of Veterinary Medicine, Dr. Bill Tranquilli has remarked, to treat an animal in pain with an unproven therapy (e.g., massage) when there exists a proven method of doing so (e.g., opiates) is immoral, because the risk that the unproven therapy will not work and that the animal will suffer outweighs the potential benefit. Even using a therapy that may have *some* potential efficacy but that displaces another that is already known to be more effective and appropriate to the animal's condition is wrong. Animals should be given the best care available.

Thus, given that the socially established concept of a veterinarian or physician is as someone who prescribes empirically validated diagnostics and therapeutics, it is wrong to violate this until such time as society acts to replace the concept with another one. The fact that members of society now ask for unproven therapies doesn't mean that they are entitled to them from scientific practitioners, who are conceptually and morally obliged to fulfill the conditions society has chartered their careers under, any more than the fact that because many farmers demanded antibiotics for growth promotion entailed that veterinarians should have acquiesced to that demand. However, if the time came that society as a whole obliterated the distinction between evidence- iand non-evidence-based medicine, the situation would involve a whole new set of rules, which is the situation next explored.

HISTORICAL ASPECTS

Today's concept of special status for medical professionals, human and veterinary, is relatively recent. Historically, competing approaches to diagnosis and therapy coexisted uneasily, with none enjoying any privileged social status. In the early nineteenth century, for example, historians tell us that there were at least two dozen varied approaches to medicine engaged in fierce competition for patients, creating a situation analogous to Thomas Hobbes's "state of nature" in the absence of government, characterized by a "war of each against all." These medical modalities included the "heroic" medicine characterized by bleeding and purging, homeopathic medicine, botanical medicine, hydropathic medicine, herbalism, and faith and folk healing. None were solidly science or evidence based. As a result, even as late as 1892, the great surgeon William Osler was still championing bleeding,[1] arguably the longest-lived of all therapies.

In a superb study of nineteenth-century medicine before the domination of the field by evidence-based, scientifically trained physicians, K. Patrick Ober has argued that the proliferation of medical modalities was to an extent a reflection of Jacksonian democracy and its bias against special privilege. Ober points out that legislative favoring of any approach to medicine was seen as limiting choice and as what today would perhaps be called "classism." According to Ober, "control of medical licensure by state legislatures had almost disappeared by 1850, and the resultant 'free trade in medicine' allowed anyone to practice medicine, regardless of qualification or training. . . . It was legal for *any citizen* of Maryland to charge for medical attention services. . . . The result was medical anarchy."

Such medical anarchy was in fact defended staunchly by many ethico-political thinkers. As Ober points out, at one stage of his life Samuel Clemens, writing as Mark Twain, defended medical anarchy:

> The mania for giving the Government power to meddle with the private affairs of cities or citizens is likely to cause endless trouble, through the rivalry of schools and creeds that are anxious to obtain official recognition, and there is great danger that our people will lose that independence of thought and action which is the cause of much of our greatness, and sink into the helplessness of the Frenchman or German who expects his government to feed him when hungry, clothe him when naked, to prescribe when his child may be born and when he may die, and, in fine, to regulate every act of humanity from the cradle to the tomb, including the manner in which he may seek future admission to paradise.[2]

Although not discussed by Ober, that reluctance to regulate was further buttressed by the successful proliferation of Adam Smith laissez-faire economics of free enterprise and the classical liberalism of Mill, both of which argued that whether in the marketplace or the marketplace of ideas, unrestricted competition was the way to wealth or truth. With the operation of the Invisible Hand of competition, wealth would emerge and truth would prevail.

In many ways, this is an attractive position. Why not let the market decide? Why not trust the citizenry to sort out what works from what doesn't work in medicine as we do in other aspects of life?

The answer has to do with knowledge and risk. People do let the market decide with regard to goods like ice cream cones and baseball bats, and services like travel booking. If the ice cream is not good, people won't buy it; if the service is defective, people will go elsewhere. However, in such situations, people are able to easily evaluate the quality and value of the goods and services they receive; such goods and services are not beyond their understanding or experience. Nor are such services administered under duress, nor are they represented as necessary for one's health or well-being (with the possible exception of ice cream).

But in the area of medicine, too much is at stake. If one chooses the wrong therapeutic modality, one can lose health, life, and limb. Furthermore, few individuals are sufficiently wealthy, educated, or possessed of the resources to test putative medical therapies. In fact, there are so many putative therapies, that it is impossible for an individual to try them all. When people are ill, they do not have the time to test even a handful. Thus, the responsibility for providing good care falls from the shoulders of the consumer (*caveat emptor*) to the shoulders of the provider (*caveat vendor*). Funding the research necessary for testing therefore falls to well-funded organizations, or governments, which have the resources to promote the large-scale testing no individual can perform.

With the development and refinement of scientific testing during the twentieth century, society and government have awarded a place of pride to science-based, empirical methodologies, and to the therapeutic modalities that pass science-based testing. As Ober demonstrates, eventually even Mark Twain relinquished his anarchical approach to medicine in favor of science-based approaches, though he continued to defend alternatives as a valuable way of keeping scientific medicine from growing arrogant and complacent.

All of this notwithstanding, anarchism continues to hold real appeal for Americans, especially when "Big Government" is widely seen as increasingly intruding into all aspects of people's lives in a heavy-handed fashion, whether in the area of sex education or suppression of medication. Resentment at government intervention in daily lives arises with regularity, as when, at the behest of the medical community, the government blocks terminally ill, suffering patients from receiving narcotics for fear of addiction or when the formula for Bronkaids, a tried and true over-the-counter remedy for asthma, was forced to change by federal government mandate on the grounds that some people were using the drug as a stimulant. People increasingly resent when the government masks highly debatable ethical choices such as the examples just enumerated as "science-based," and issues decisions that affect individuals on the basis of ethics masquerading as science.

In today's world it is easy to share the anarchist view that government and its ever-proliferating bureaucracy are sources of problems, not of solutions. It is hard not to feel that oftentimes people could work out their own problems absent the ham-fisted touch of government, corporations, or other large organizations.

Cooperation and mutual interdependence without government intervention is anarchism in the classical nineteenth-century sense. As such, it was argued that the presence of authority creates distance across people, whereas its absence and the mutual interdependence that it creates militates in favor of people caring for one another. Thus, it is not surprising that a spark of anarchism burns in many Americans, and that this spark may manifest itself in part in a defiance of government-supported medicine or large medical organizations (such as the AVMA). Add beliefs that government "screws that up the way it screws up everything else" and even conspiratorial theories, such as the contention that the government wants to block access to viable therapies, and a sympathetic alternative underdog may arise.

MEDICAL ANARCHISM

Probably the most brilliant and articulate voice for an anarchistic approach to science and medicine in the twentieth century is the late German philosopher Paul Feyerabend. In an erudite series of books and articles, Feyerabend explored the incompatibility of scientific hegemony with true democracy.[3] Feyerabend points out that most people would be prepared to admit that science prevails as the government-supported way of knowing and approaching problems, be the issues medical or environmental or agricultural, because, as was said earlier, science *works*. People predict and control the world they live in best if they put science and technology at the basis of their social decision making, not Navajo shamanism. Science gives people the most power over nature, therefore science works best.

Feyerabend's key insight, overlooked by most, is that what counts as "working" or, more clearly, working *best*, is a judgment of value, rather than a mere judgment of fact. And if this is the case, science only works better than other approaches when assessed by the criteria built into science, for example assuming that "predicting and controlling" is always more desirable than "living in harmony with."

As an example, many agricultural scientists would say that the development of intensive agriculture through science is the best agriculture society could have because such agriculture results in greater productivity and efficiency. Indeed, agricultural scientists are so wedded to these values at the expense of all others, that they see anyone critical of intensive agriculture as ungrateful or even sinful. Yet where is this written? Why can't a rational person condemn science-based intensive agriculture on the grounds of its lack of sustainability, its consumption of resources, its despoliation of the environment, its destruction of animal husbandry, or its major contribution to the demise of rural communities? Is it irrational to reject greater productivity if it comes at a cost of irreparable damage to the values underlying sustainability, husbandry, and community? Is it irrational to prefer environmental health to ridiculously cheap food? Surely not, and one can further argue that cheap and plentiful food has led to dietary lifestyles that damage health!

To encounter a true Feyerabendian is to find one's taken-for-granted values seriously challenged, indeed struck by lightning. A Navajo student who had a degree in public health from Harvard and was completing an animal science degree provided some interesting perspective. Due to her minority standing, the world was her oyster. "What are you going to do now?" she was asked. "Med school? A PhD in biological science? Molecular biology?"

"No" she said quietly. "I am going back to the reservation to help my grand-mother tend her sheep."

"What?" she was asked incredulously. "Are you going to waste all that education? Throw away all your opportunities? Trash everything?"

"Let me put it this way," she said. "At Harvard and Colorado State University I learned the biological explanation for a ewe's having twin lambs. As a child, my grandmother taught me that twin lambs were a reward from the animal for good husbandry. I prefer the latter."

I prefer the latter. Feyerabend's point is hereby made, namely that it is possible to understand and know science and the scientific worldview, yet prefer an alternate one!

This point can also be illustrated with a medical example. Suppose someone suffers from terminal cancer. For a variety of reasons that have been discussed previously, science-based physicians will largely work to prolong that person's life, regardless of the qualitative deteriorative changes in that life—the suffering associated with radical surgery or chemotherapy, the emotional cost to that person and his or her family, the financial cost, the suffering, and so on. If, in the process, that person gets pneumonia, scientific physicians will attempt to cure it, perhaps gaining an extra few months of agonized existence. Would it be irrational to prefer, as one finds in hospice, a less technological, less science-based approach to terminal illness that concentrates on dying with dignity, controlling suffering, surrounding you at the end with those who care about you; that views pneumonia, as people did when they could not cure it, as "the old person's friend" because it took life gently as people simply faded?

Feyerabend's point is that there are innumerable systems of value that reject science's belief that prediction and control of nature is the *summum bonum*. The Navajo shaman would rather live in harmony with nature than control it, accept the inevitable rather than forever be at war with it. That represents a different position but not necessarily a stupid or irrational one .

Further, argues Feyerabend, society is inherently pluralistic in culture and value. Why should social decision-making bodies be peopled exclusively by scientists who would rather spend billions of dollars on research into disease than on educating the poor? Why does a president's commission on the environment consist largely of scientists, not of shamans? If in a truly free and democratic society, why do the values of science permeate all decision making? Why is the money of those inimical to science spent supporting science? Why not let subcultures choose their own ways of knowing as they chose their own religions? Why doesn't a teleological biology that is based in aesthetic appreciation of the beauty of interrelated functions in nature receive as much funding as mechanistic molecular biology?

WHY GIVE MEDICINE SPECIAL PRIVILEGES?

Thus emerges a very philosophically sophisticated version of Samuel Clemens's medical anarchy: Why give hegemony to science and evidence-based medical practitioners, why afford them special privileges, why not remove official social support from all approaches to medicine, and let people decide for themselves? For this is surely the logical consequence of the practitioners, human and animal, whom society has charged with guarding the gates of medicine and assuring that therapies and diagnostics are evidence based, dabbling with and admixing non-evidence-based therapies into putatively scientific medicine. If no medical approach is special, why give social priority to *any* group of practitioners?

Given the significant increase in social demand for alternative medicine (now estimated at 29 billion dollars per year), should the Feyerabendian model prevail? Should there be no social sanctioning of any one approach to medicine but simply establish "anything goes"?

It seems likely that in the views of most physicians, veterinarians, and members of the public, the answer is still a resounding "No!" For, as argued in chapter 3, people still wish to give primacy to what medicine *works* in a demonstrably curative or palliative sense. What works is still almost universally believed to be what can stand up to objective scrutiny, that is, meet the tests of scientific validation. Since there are far more approaches to medical therapy than anyone can individually test, people want quality control performed at some level.

In addition to science-based or validated approaches to therapy, there exist countless others. These include not only long-established traditions of currently popular cultures such as the Chinese, but also a ragtag myriad others, some of which are based in religious views, shamanistic views, well-developed systems of magic, demonology, and so on. Suppose a medical professional is being asked to treat a tumor. If every established and even every promising experimental therapeutic modality has been exhausted, if the patient, human or animal, can be offered no more evidence-based therapies, given the mission to heal, the patient and the professional may now be approached by the myriad other non-science-based modalities claiming to be efficacious. What principle of selection is employed in order to decide what to try next? Should the patient purchase a ticket to Lourdes because there are countless anecdotal attestations concerning the miraculous efficacy of the waters? Or should the patient go to the Philippines to receive psychic surgery? After all, there's a *possibility* that an effective psychic surgeon may be encountered, even though all of them evaluated to date have been exposed as frauds. Or does the doctor recommend that the patient go through demonological approaches, which come highly recommended by centuries of anecdotal attestation, or investigate the power of prayer, for which there are vast numbers of testimonials?

The point is that once a medical practitioner has abandoned a scientific empirical basis for recommending therapies, there is nothing to stand in its stead as a basis for making recommendations. Furthermore, there is no basis by which harm can be reasonably avoided. Patients and owners have neither unlimited time nor unlimited resources, so one must narrow the options. How then, does one do so without controlled testing? In other words, "anything goes" anarchic medicine does nothing to sift the possibilities for patients. This is indeed why scientific medicine has gained ascendance; it does provide a criterion acceptable to most people for sifting through countless possible therapies—testability and repeatability and the others discussed in an earlier chapter. As soon as physicians or veterinarians abandon these criteria, they have ceased to practice as society has chartered them to practice, that is, to offer up therapies that are evidence based. As such, they have ceased to objectively search for effective therapies.

ABANDONING RESPONSIBILITY

Nevertheless, it is easy to see how abandonment of this responsibility occurs despite the solid scientific basis for medicine required of licensed practitioners. First of all, science does not know everything. Second, people in medicine confuse two conceptually distinct roles: the role of evidence-based therapist and diagnostician for which they are specially trained and licensed, and the far more nebulous and ancient role of healer. Even when scientific medicine has exhausted therapeutic options, medical people still wish to heal their patients! This is further invigorated by the fact that physicians and veterinarians *are* venerated as healers and thereby possess significant Aesculapian authority to shape people's behavior, get them to change lifestyle, validate periods of rest or absence from work responsibility, and even on occasion to get one to feel better in their presence! Such a role is heady stuff for one who assumes it.

Though it is sometimes psychologically difficult to separate one's role as healer from one's role as medical professional, the two are conceptually distinct.

As veterinarians or physicians, individuals are licensed by society to deal with disease, illness, and disability, according to the modalities of diagnosis and treatment established by the scientific basis of biomedicine. Individuals are constrained—or should be constrained—within those confines. As healers, individuals may yearn for other modalities, yet to deploy them can bring down social ire in the form of malpractice judgments. Licensed professionals are first and foremost science- and evidence-based practitioners. No matter how much they believe personally in the water of Lourdes, they cannot write prescriptions for it; no matter how much they believe in healing by prayer, they cannot employ prayer as a therapeutic modality. All this follows from society's desire to avoid medical chaos, rank therapies as more or less proven or evidence based, and have science-trained practitioners serve as gatekeepers or guardians of quality control. No matter the size of the expenditure on unproven alternatives, it does not prove that society wants its gatekeepers to venture far beyond the boundaries it has set for them. Indeed, it far more proves the power of wishful thinking.

The desire to be a healer is a good desire, but it is seductive, and it can be channeled incorrectly if it leads one to embrace nonscientific therapies. This seems to be the consensus emerging in human medical journals about physicians invoking religion to help them heal patients. That is, instead of medical practitioners embracing the role of healer by moving toward untested therapies, it makes far more sense for them to acknowledge and respond to the concerns we outlined in previous chapters, that is, to place more emphasis on the patient's individuality, more emphasis on pain and suffering and other modes of subjectivity that scientific ideology has suppressed, and more emphasis on genuine dialogue with the patient.

In veterinary medicine, there is less obvious room to relate to the patient as an individual, though there is certainly *some* room to do so, and certainly more room to emphasize comfort, care rather than cure. At the same time, there is greater risk of straying from a rational path in veterinary medicine since (1) clients, not patients, foot the bill and, (2) unlike the case of children, society has not yet determined a sufficient moral status for animals for them to be direct objects of moral concern and medical attention.

A parent, who, in lieu of validated therapeutic methods, insisted on colored light or prayer therapy for a child's trauma, would be corrected by the legal system; this is not true for an animal! Since animals are legally considered property, owners can, by and large, dictate whatever therapies they choose. There are even reports of veterinarians who claim to talk to the spirits of animals and whom clients consult for guidance on euthanasia when the animal is very ill. If the spirit says it is not ready to go, the client will withhold euthanasia regardless of how much the animal is suffering. *Perhaps* such a tack could in principle be challenged under the anticruelty laws as failing to provide adequate veterinary care, but who would lead such an action? At any rate, such a case would probably be denied by the courts, which tend to be conservative regarding cruelty and therefore are reluctant to prosecute anyone but those in whom cruelty to animals is clearly a sentinel for potential abuse of humans.

MORAL OBLIGATIONS

Most veterinarians, when asked the fundamental question of veterinary ethics, "To whom do you have primary moral obligation, owner or animal?" unhesitatingly reply, "The animal." Certainly, the public image of the veterinarian is based on this assumption, and veterinarians would almost certainly not wish to lose that image. However, if that is the case, then the primary function of a veterinarian is to benefit his or her charges, not satisfy owners. And it is clearly noncontroversial that a proven therapy trumps one that remains to be proven. Thus, the vulnerability of the animal and the veterinarian's role together militate in favor of proven therapy rather than untested therapy at least where these notions have meaning. This augments the earlier point that the public at large still wishes a winnowing of therapies by way of experts who know where evidence lies.

Further, it also seems obvious that most veterinarians who do recommend alternative therapies are not seeking an "anything goes" anarchistic model for medical services. Few practitioners, like few members of society, would wish to see all possible therapies treated equally. As in ethics, no one truly and reflectively believes that one's choices are simply a matter of opinion. Rather, those practitioners may be asserting that the scientific community has exerted a stranglehold on what gets looked at or is taken seriously as a potential therapy. That is, they may be concerned that some therapies derived from other medical traditions are being given short shrift. (In his less anarchistic moments, this seems to be what Feyerabend claims.) In other words, the argument is not that there are alternative methods for establishing that therapies work as curative or palliative, but rather that scientific medicine has systematically excluded certain therapies, for which there is some prima facie or even significant evidence of efficacy, from serious empirical testing for arbitrary reasons, such as place of origin.

This argument can be viewed sympathetically. Anyone who studies the history of science knows that science has its own prejudices, on occasion, even bigotries. Consider Einstein's remark, made after reporters learned that Eddington's astronomical observations had confirmed the General Theory of Relativity. Einstein was asked what he would have said had the data not done so. "So much the worse for the data," he replied. "The theory is correct." Similarly, Harlow Shapley of the Hayden Planetarium roundly condemned Velikovsky's cosmological book *Worlds in Collision*. When reporters grilled

Shapley as to specific examples from the book that represented egregious errors, Shapley replied freely that he could give no examples, not having in fact read the book. In another telling example, a well-known physiologist confided that he had been extremely fortunate in receiving research funding. In fact, he said, the only time he has ever had a proposal turned down was when, if his thesis proved to be correct, the research would cast doubt on the dominant paradigm, adhered to by everyone deciding on his funding!

Hostility to certain approaches may arise from powerful theoretical commitments that exclude a given medical approach and create what has been called "paradigm blindness." Alternative approaches may also be threatening to established individuals and be met with much initial skepticism. In one notable recent example from medicine, it was proposed that gastric ulcers were caused by an infection with *H. pylori*. Despite initial criticism, this proposal turned out to be correct in some cases. The Catholic Church met Galileo's astronomic observations with derision and contempt. Of course, in both examples, it was subsequent experimentation and replication that validated the initial observations.

However, the knife of prejudice cuts both ways. Proscience biases may clash with more liberal approaches on the other side. The person open to acupuncture may cite its allegedly successful use for centuries in the Orient and be satisfied that this is *a priori* evidence that acupuncture is effective. However, such open-mindedness may overlook the fact that numerous ineffective therapies and approaches have been used for much longer time periods—*vide* astrology or therapeutic bleeding—and still be open to disproof. Merely because an idea is *not* part of the established paradigm, has been subjected to ridicule by the "establishment," or has been around for a long time does not also mean that it is valid—as Carl Sagan noted, "They laughed at Galileo, but they also laughed at Bozo the Clown."

Medical science has been highly selective in what it chooses to examine as possibly efficacious, and has generally ignored the medical traditions of radically different cultures. (Interestingly enough, drug companies are nowhere near as xenophobic as academicians in their willingness to look at primitive societies' medicaments when they dispatch ethnobotanists and ethnopharmacologists.) It seems reasonable to suggest that any sophisticated and long-lived society possessed of an intricate and complex culture would evolve remedies worth examining, and would certainly be worth examining for historical interest. China certainly fits this description; so does India; so do the virtually ignored traditions of Islamic medicine. But again, therapeutic approaches derived from other cultures should not be presumed efficacious by virtue of their longevity, rather, they may be plausible candidates for scientific testing, testing that has not been forthcoming in the past.

Thus, if the argument is that therapies arising from other cultures should be tested, not ignored, there is no quarrel with science. Indeed, it makes sense to test plants that very primitive societies have used to treat ailments before testing plants at random. But this is *not* to presume that such remedies are efficacious in the absence of standard scientific testing.

In the same vein, remedies for which there is much anecdotal support might also be reasonable candidates for submission to scientific testing. However, such anecdotes should not be grounds for establishing the efficacy of a remedy—as previously noted, there are numerous reasons why ineffective remedies might be perceived to be effective. Furthermore, if the underlying rationale for the therapies is at odds with well-established fact, the chances that such therapies will prove ultimately useful are remote. At best, strong anecdotal support should be a reason to jump the putative modality to the front of the testing line.

ALTERNATIVES TO MEDICAL SCIENCE

The alternative to establishing science-based practitioners as the socially accepted filterers of medical therapies is medical anarchy. However, while such anarchism is in some respects attractive on its face, it is ultimately unacceptable for a variety of reasons. It would leave no rational decision procedure for choosing among competing therapies. Society, on reflection, is unlikely to want such a state of therapeutic anarchism. Veterinarians would almost certainly not want it because their legal status as primary caregivers for animals would be adversely affected. In addition, veterinary medical anarchy could and would create much animal suffering, given the property status of animals and the sovereignty of owners. Nonetheless, the anarchist critique legitimately points out the bias that has resided in the science-based medical community against testing remedies established in other cultures. It would be prudent to test these therapies scientifically as soon as possible, if only to dispel the notion of a conspiracy against them, though their longevity should not count as evidence for their efficacy.

9

Regulatory Considerations

Discussions of therapeutic efficacy, scientific evidence, and ethics aside, the fact is that CAVM approaches challenge standard veterinary medicine. As such, they have clamored for, and received, much attention. To the extent that such clamor can uncover new and useful therapies, or push some practitioners to listen to the concerns of their clients, the debate is likely to be of ultimate benefit to animals and veterinarians. However, one must be mindful of the "law of unintended consequences." The ancient Chinese initially developed a mixture of saltpeter (potassium nitrate), sulfur, and charcoal or dry honey as a treatment for skin diseases and as a fumigant to kill insects. In A.D. 850, this formula, which came to be known as gunpowder, was published in a book called *Classified Essentials of the Mysterious Tao of the True Origin of Things*. The author warned that "smoke and flames result, so that [the experimenters'] hands and faces have been burned, and even the whole house where they were working burned down." The deadly potential of gunpowder soon found a use in unintended ways. So it is with CAVM, which threatens to burn down the exclusive therapeutic house in which veterinarians have been residing.[1]

IS REGULATION OF CAVM WISE?

It is inarguable that the promises of CAVM appeal to some clients, if for no other reason than because such practices may offer psychological support to those attempting to confront an animal's various ills (real or perceived). However, veterinary professionals should be mindful that psychosocial support, no matter how important, is not the unique purview of their profession.

Attempting to restrict the practice of every single conceivable modality to veterinarians has the potential for making veterinarians look like bullies trying to pick on the new kids in the neighborhood. Virtually anyone can provide emotional support in times of crisis. Attempts to regulate such support would seem to be futile—indeed, they might rather be viewed as shortsighted, as they might induce conflict between the professional and client and force the client to choose between a compassionate layperson and a veterinarian who is perceived as having "poor bedside manner." It might behoove the profession to consider giving more attention to the psychological interactions that occur between doctor and client (the art of medicine), however, this is not the purview of science, nor of regulation. Rather, it should be part of education in veterinary-client-patient interactions.

That said, regulation of veterinary medicine cannot concern itself merely with psychosocial interactions. Effective therapies can be delivered in a gruff and insensitive fashion; ineffective remedies can be delivered with compassion. Effective regulation of medical practices can only be attempted based on objective criteria of efficacy.

HOW PREVALENT IS THE USE OF ALTERNATIVE MEDICINE?

Recent surveys in human medicine reveal that the use of alternative modalities by human patients is considerably less than has been previously reported. Most recently, an analysis of data from the 1999 National Health Interview Survey (NHIS), covering the 30,801 respondents of the noninstitutionalized civilian population of the United States, ages 18 and older, found that an estimated 28.9 percent of U.S. adults used at least one CAM therapy in the previous year. The three most commonly used therapies were spiritual healing or prayer (13.7 percent)[2], herbal medicine (9.6 percent), and chiropractic therapies (7.6 percent). Acupuncture was used by 1.7 percent of the population surveyed and homeopathy by 3.1 percent. Interestingly, alternative medicine use was generally in addition to, rather than instead of, scientific medicine.[3] Clearly, alternative medicine has not convinced its users of the superiority of its approach, nor does it appear to be judged as an alternative to mainstream medicine by its users. Accordingly, it does not seem obvious that radical changes in regulatory standards or in educational curriculums need to be made in an effort to accommodate a distinct minority of the population that uses or applies alternative therapies.

In veterinary medicine, surveys of CAVM use by clients appear to be virtually nonexistent. A 2000 survey on educational and research programs in CAVM by United States veterinary schools noted that a distinct minority of the veterinary colleges offers classes in CAVM, and none has a required course or is proposing one.[4] A 2000 survey of member hospitals conducted by the American Animal Hospital Association (AAHA) found that the number of individuals using CAVM is actually quite small. Sixty-nine percent of the survey respondents reported using no alternative modalities at all, a mere 3 percent used acupuncture, and another 2 percent used veterinary chiropractic.[5]

WHAT IS THE CURRENT STATE OF REGULATION OF PRACTITIONERS OF ALTERNATIVE MEDICINE ON HUMANS?

Obviously, the current state of any regulation is in a state of flux. In particular, the necessity for—and ideal type of—regulation of alternative medical practices is the subject of fierce debate, both in veterinary and human medicine. As such, new regulations and modifications of existing ones seem to be appearing continually. Furthermore, there is wide variation among the regulations of individual states. Thus, to be assured of accuracy in particular circumstances, interested individuals should check with the regulations of their individual jurisdictions prior to instituting therapy.

Acupuncture

At this time, approximately 40 states of the United States have put in place some form of surveillance regulation pertaining to human acupuncture. However, less than 50 percent of those identify any need for *undergraduate* education. Most states do not require any biomedical knowledge for the practice of acupuncture. The primary requirement for recognition is the completion of a state-approved acupuncture course, although a few states recognize apprenticeship training as adequate. The National Commission for the Certification of Acupuncture and Oriental Medicine provides the course accepted by most states. It comprises 1,725 hours (most veterinary programs offer less than one-tenth of that).

Some states deem that acupuncture is medical practice, and the medical boards of about 12 states thereby provide surveillance. However, MDs and doctors of osteopathy in 31 other states can practice acupuncture without any certification whatsoever. Still other states direct that physicians who practice acupuncture must have the same training as nonphysicians in the field. In 3 states, chiropractors can practice acupuncture with no training at all, while 7 require 100 hours of training.[6]

Chiropractic

The number of chiropractic institutions in the United States is stable, and all except one are privately funded. Nearly 50 percent of the students who enter chiropractic colleges do so with a baccalaureate degree. Chiropractic colleges require that students receive four years of education, and upon graduation, they can apply for licensure examinations. Forty-six states either recognize or require passage of examinations given by the National Board of Chiropractic Examiners before granting a license to practice. Most states require annual proof of continuing education for license renewal.[7]

Homeopathy

Currently, the practice of homeopathy is largely unregulated in the United States. As of 2003, three states (Arizona, Connecticut, and Nevada) license homeopathic practice for physicians already licensed in that state.

Herbal and Botanical Medicine

The practice of herbal and botanical medicine currently appears to be largely unregulated in the United States. This is in large part due to the Dietary Supplement Health and Education Act of 1994 (DSHEA), which limited the role of the Food and Drug Administration (FDA) in regulating such products. In doing so, DSHEA essentially deregulated the herb and dietary supplements industry, and created an economic boom. Under the act, herbal medications are held to a lesser standard than prescription drugs. The animal investigations, clinical trials, and postmarketing surveillance that are *de rigeur* for pharmaceutical products are not required for herbal or other supplement preparations intended for human consumption. In addition, removing an herbal or supplement product from the market is difficult and requires that the FDA show "convincing evidence" of adverse effects.

The myriad herbal concoctions, with inconsistent compositions and inadequate quality control, have turned out to be a regulatory nightmare for overseeing agencies. Over a five-year span (1993–1998), approximately 2,600 adverse events and one hundred deaths associated with dietary supplements were reported to the FDA.[8] No central mechanism for mandatory reporting of such adverse effects exists, so the actual incidence is unknown. The resulting underreporting further limits the amount of information the FDA can accrue when it considers building a case for regulation of a particular herbal product or supplement. Therefore, the FDA is constrained to be reactive rather than proactive in limiting the sale of potentially toxic herbal substances.[9] As a result, anarchy has replaced regulation in an area where government should and must be responsible for verifying safety and efficacy.

Other Alternative Modalities

Licensing bodies exist for the practice of massage in most states. At least 11 states license naturopaths, with varying requirements. For example, the requirements for licensing in the state of Oregon are graduation from an approved school of naturopathy (certified by the Board of Naturopathy: currently four naturopaths and one citizen representative) and passing a licensing test.

WHAT IS VETERINARY MEDICINE?

In most states, veterinary medicine is defined broadly, presumably in an attempt to limit the practice of providing animal health care services to veterinarians or those who are directly supervised by veterinarians. With these definitions as a guide, veterinary medicine is generally considered a way to "diagnosis, treat, correct, change, relieve, or prevent animal disease, deformity, defect, injury, or other physical or mental condition" using any number of techniques and devices.[10] In general, these techniques and devices also include CAVM therapies, such as acupuncture, veterinary chiropractic (also referred to as manual therapy or manipulation), homeopathy, and even magnetic therapy.[11] This situation is somewhat unique to veterinary medicine; in human alternative therapies, statutory protection is generally not given to human medical doctors from providers of alternative therapies to humans. Thus, it should not be assumed that the situation cannot change in veterinary medicine.

WHAT IS THE STATE OF REGULATION OF VETERINARIANS OFFERING CAVM?

In some states, veterinary practice acts have been or are being changed to specifically refer to CAVM. For example, in 1999, the state of Oklahoma amended its definition of the "practice of veterinary medicine" specifically to include alternative medicine,[12] and it defined alternative medicine as "a variety of therapeutic philosophies, tools, and treatment approaches to veterinary health care delivery, consisting of biochemical, biomechanical, bioenergetic and lifestyle therapies, which include but are not limited to acupuncture and acutherapy, chiropractic, physical therapy, massage therapy, homeopathy, botanical medicine, nutraceutical medicine and holistic medicine."

Rather than strictly limit the practice of working on animals to veterinarians, some state veterinary boards have developed rules or policy statements in an attempt to clarify when a veterinarian can call in a nonlicensed individual (such as a chiropractor or acupuncturist) to treat an animal. For example, in 1998, the state of California penned specific regulations pertaining to "musculoskeletal manipulation" of animals. This was an attempt to let chiropractors practice on animals under direct veterinary supervision.[13] Other states have followed a similar approach and have tried to allow virtually any therapy to be used, and for that therapy to be applied by any person, so long as that therapy is applied under direct supervision by a veterinarian.[14] The most detailed regulations on the use of CAVM therapies currently appear to be those of the state of Texas.[15]

WHAT IS THE CURRENT STATUS OF REGULATION REGARDING PRACTITIONERS OF ALTERNATIVE HUMAN MEDICINE ON ANIMALS?

Most alternative human therapists, such as chiropractors and/or acupuncturists, are generally restrained by law from practicing on animals, because many state acupuncture and/or chiropractic acts specifically refer to humans.[16] As was noted, the practice of veterinary medicine is generally limited to veterinarians by state statute. This works both ways. For example, in the state of Ohio, it is not permissible for a veterinarian to advertise using the term *chiropractic care*, *animal chiropractor*, or *chiropractic* unless he or she is a licensed doctor of chiropractic. This distinction is also noted in the 2001 AVMA Guidelines on the use of CAVM therapies. The guidelines take note of the fact that chiropractic is generally defined as being practiced on humans, and thus refers to such manipulations as *manual therapy*. That term, in turn, has been adopted by Colorado State University for its continuing education course.

Under any circumstances, it is perhaps naïve to think that the current state of affairs might not change. Indeed, challenges to the veterinary practice acts have been forthcoming and should be expected to arise with increasing regularity. For example, in 1994, Maryland's Acupuncture Act was amended by the Maryland Legislature to delete the word *human* from the definition section of the act.[17] Then, in 1995, Maryland's attorney general issued a legal opinion stating that acupuncturists in Maryland could perform acupuncture on animals without being licensed veterinarians.[18] Although the Maryland attorney general's opinion was that animal acupuncture fell under the legal definition of the state statutes pertaining to the practice of veterinary medicine under the Maryland Veterinary Practice Act, he also noted that the Maryland Acupuncture Board had authority over the practice of acupuncture. Thus, he concluded that "if, under the *Maryland Acupuncture Act*, the activity of performing acupuncture on an animal falls within the scope of the practice of acupuncture, a licensee of the Acupuncture Board may practice animal acupuncture, although the very same activity is also within the scope of the practice of veterinary medicine." Following the Maryland attorney general's opinion, the Maryland legislature then changed Maryland's Veterinary Practice Act to allow *any* acupuncturist to treat animals, subject to some regulation.[19] Some of the most vigorous objections to the change in the law came from veterinary acupuncturists, who asserted that a veterinary education was necessary to protect animals from acupuncture, "inappropriately" applied. However, such arguments did not hold sway. Since acupuncture is inherently nonscientific, having been developed centuries before scientific standards of inquiry, and it lacks evidence for efficacy, it may be difficult to show what is the most appropriate way to apply it.

On the other hand, on June 5, 1998, the Michigan Court of Appeals overruled a decision of the Michigan Board of Chiropractic and reinstated a cease and desist order of the Michigan Department of Consumer & Industry Services. In that order, the Michigan department stated that a chiropractor performing services on animals without a veterinary license or under the supervision of a licensed veterinarian was engaged in unlawful practice of veterinary medicine.[20] Undaunted by such setbacks, chiropractors appear to be particularly interested in changing the veterinary practice acts. For example, the state of Wisconsin proposed legislation (LRB 4138) that would have created a separate certification to practice as an animal chiropractor in Wisconsin. Furthermore, the bill would have permitted unlicensed individuals, such as chiropractors, to diagnose and treat animals without a veterinary referral. In Nevada, Senate Bill 510 would have amended the state's chiropractic laws to allow a DC, who is certified by the American Veterinary Chiropractic Association and also licensed in Nevada, to perform animal chiropractic "without the order, referral, direction or supervision of a person who is licensed as a veterinarian." As such, the bill would have changed the veterinary laws in Nevada to remove "chiropractic procedures" from the definition of "practice of veterinary medicine." It would have thereby prevented the veterinary board from regulating individuals performing animal chiropractic. In fact, this position is explicitly supported by the American Veterinary Chiropractic Association, which wants veterinary chiropractic regulated as a profession separate and distinct from veterinary medicine.

Pressure comes from other areas, as well. For example, calls for the entry of chiropractic into the veterinary field have been published in professional chiropractic journals.[21] In a similar vein, the orthopedic section of the American Physical Therapy Association has formed an Animal Physical Therapist Special Interest Group to "explore new fields of practice."[22] Finally, in 2003, in the state of Connecticut, a bill was proposed recommending that the general statutes be changed to "exclude myofascial trigger point therapy performed by persons experienced in such therapy from the definition of the practice of veterinary medicine."[23]

Certification?

Practitioners of the various CAVM modalities may or may not choose to be certified in their particular area of interest. Still, it is not necessarily clear what expertise such certification entails. Any number of organizations grant certification, and a veterinary degree may or may not be required to gain it. Currently, there are

1. At least three groups that certify veterinary acupuncturists (International Veterinary Acupuncture Society, Chi Institute, and the American Academy of Veterinary Medical Acupuncture at Colorado State University).

2. At least two courses granting certification in veterinary chiropractic or manual therapy (American Veterinary Chiropractic Association, Colorado State University). The AVCA also certifies doctors of chiropractic to adjust animals. One-day courses in veterinary chiropractic are offered by Daniel Kamen, DC, a doctor of chiropractic, author of the "Well Adjusted" series of animal books. Dr. Kamen's courses are open to anyone. Further certification in veterinary orthopedic manipulation is also offered.*

3. At least one organization grants certification in veterinary homeopathy, the Academy of Veterinary Homeopathy, although classes leading to certification may be taught by other individuals. Online certificates in homeopathy may also be obtained.[24]

4. Continuing education classes in herbal and botanical medicine are offered by Colorado State University (with primary instruction being given by a nonveterinarian). Certification is offered by the Veterinary Botanical Medicine Association, both to veterinarians as certified veterinary herbalists and to laypeople as certified veterinary herbalism educators.

5. A variety of classes and schools certifies massage therapists.

6. Certification in the application of numerous modalities such as low-intensity lasers and electroacuscopes may be available from the manufacturers or developers of those modalities.

Unfortunately, from a regulatory standpoint, certification in *any* CAVM modality means very little. Certification in any CAVM modality certainly does

---

*http://www.peaceofmindvet.com/vom.html: "VOM [veterinary orthopedic manipulation] exists between veterinary medicine and chiropractic care. It has similarities to human chiropractic modalities and functions by reducing subluxations. It employs a hand-held device that is used in human chiropractic, Activator Methods; but it is not to be confused with that technique. Activator Methods, developed by Arlan Fuhr, D.C., uses the spinal accelerometer but relies on listings, which are anatomical subluxation signs demonstrated by leg length checks. VOM is also not manual adjusting as taught by the American Veterinary Chiropractic Association (AVCA). VOM is a gentle and safe method of reducing subluxations. The American Veterinary Medical Association (AVMA) does not recognize veterinary chiropractic care (VOM or AVCA) for now. The American Holistic Veterinary Medical Association formally recognizes VOM."

not imply that the modality in question has therapeutic benefit, nor does such certification reflect any recognized objective standards. Rather, the requirements for certification are solely based on the opinions of the individual or individuals who are doing the certifying[†]

Nor are certified individuals necessarily the only ones who might be able to effectively practice a particular modality. For example, if one of the appeals of acupuncture is its traditional nature, it is easy to imagine that a family-educated Chinese traditional practitioner might be as well or more skilled in its application than a newly trained veterinarian. Or, one might consider that chiropractors, for whom approximately 1,500 hours of training in the various chiropractic manipulations is required, would be more qualified to apply those manipulations to animals than would be "certified" veterinarians who have much less training.

It is therefore not possible to assert which, if any, certified individual is competent to practice on an animal. Indeed, there is virtually no barrier to entry into many of the various CAVM fields—education is not a prerequisite for most of them. Accordingly, it is impossible to propose regulations based on certification. Nor can it be logically asserted that therapies for which certification exist are useful merely because of the existence of some certifying body. Such reasoning is entirely circular.

It is important to note that CAVM practices appear to be most useful in treating minor ailments (usually in those that are self-limiting), for the treatment of chronic, incurable conditions, for the treatment of well animals, or in addition to effective therapies (complementary). However, these same practices do not seem to be as useful in severe or acute conditions. The various interventions (needles, lights, magnets, manipulation of the spine, single or nonexistent atoms, and megadoses of vitamins) may be effective to treat mild fevers but not pneumonia, to treat malaise but not shock.

It may be instructive to examine the conditions for which practitioners of human alternative medicine feel their treatments are of most benefit. A 2001

[†]Steve K. D. Eichel, PhD, a practicing psychologist in Philadelphia, Pennsylvania, obtained certificates for his cat from five organizations. The only requirement was completing of an online questionnaire and payment of a fee. None checked any of the cat's alleged credentials. The cat also obtained "board certification" from two organizations. One organization asked for a copy of the cat's curriculum vitae, however, it did not ask for any documentation of credentials or check whether anything listed in the CV was genuine. Nor did it require any examination before issuing a certificate attesting to the cat having met "rigid requirements" resulting in her "designation as a Diplomate." The acceptance letter that accompanied the certificate stated that diplomate status "is limited to a select group of professionals who, by virtue of their extensive training and expertise, have demonstrated their outstanding abilities in regard to their specialty" (Eichel, S. K. D. Credentialing: It may not be the cat's meow. Greater Philadelphia Society of Clinical Hypnosis website, accessed November 14, 2002; http://users.snip.net/~drsteve/Articles/Dr_Zoe.htm).

survey in the United Kingdom evaluated exactly that. Surveys were sent to 223 organizations representing various techniques—two or more responses were sent back by representatives of 12 therapies (aromatherapy, Bach flower remedies, Bowen technique, chiropractic, homoeopathy, hypnotherapy, magnet therapy, massage, nutrition, reflexology, Reiki, and yoga). The top seven conditions amenable to the various therapies were (1) stress/anxiety, (2) headaches/migraine, (3) back pain, (4) respiratory problems (including asthma), (5) insomnia, (6) "cardiovascular problems," and (7) "musculoskeletal problems."

Exactly none of the conditions for which the therapies were advocated represented an organic cause of disease. The conditions were mostly chronic, incurable, or self-limiting, and also may have some psychological component. Furthermore, "no obvious correlation between length of training and treatment cost was apparent."[25]

What explanation is there for this? Might it be that the practices don't really work or that the putative mechanisms of action are merely nonspecific stimuli? If that's the case, perhaps there's no need for education or certification in such CAVM modalities at all. Indeed, certification seems mostly as advertisement, allowing promotion of CAVM practices to the public and implying a certain level of expertise and competence. In fact, none may exist or be necessary.

In its 2001 guidelines, the AVMA notes: "The AVMA does not officially recognize diplomate status or certificates other than those awarded by veterinary specialty organizations that are members of the AVMA American Board of Veterinary Specialties (ABVS), nor has it evaluated the training or education programs of other entities that provide such certificates. Recognition of a veterinary specialty organization by the AVMA requires demonstration of a substantial body of scientific knowledge. The AVMA encourages CAVM organizations to demonstrate such a body of knowledge." To date, no such organization has done so.

ON WHAT BASIS IS STATUTORY PROTECTION GRANTED TO VETERINARIANS?

As has been noted, societal expectations that veterinarians will apply effective therapies imply that the public expects that veterinarians will employ science-based canons of proof and evidence in evaluating and regulating diagnostic and therapeutic modalities. To be a scientific professional one must be bound by and committed to the rules and canons of science, and accept those rules as the standards for judging truth and falsity of empirical claims, including the efficacy of therapies. The dedication to scientific validation of therapies, above all other considerations, sets medical professionals apart from unlicensed individuals in the eyes of society. Without an objective standard by which therapies can be evaluated, or without a dedication to acquiring such a standard, veterinary medicine becomes a morass of separate but equal approaches in the minds of both practitioners and the public. As such, regulation becomes impossible.

REGULATORY DILEMMAS

At least seven issues are important in considering the regulatory dilemmas posed by CAVM to veterinary medicine.

1. How to Regulate Unproven Practices

With no substantive body of supporting scientific knowledge, and expertise and applications based on individual standards and preferences, it is not possible to objectively regulate the practice(s) of CAVM. Similarly, since the use of unvalidated treatment options is solely based on individual preference, it is also impossible to determine such things as minimum standards of care. Indeed, notions of standardization, appropriateness, and standard of care, which are inherent in developing and applying professional regulations, are antithetical to CAVM, which considers many different and unrelated practices as appropriate and encourages different belief systems and divergent theories about the nature of health and disease, as well as fundamental differences as to how target conditions are defined, appropriate interventions, and outcome measures of effectiveness.[26] As an example of the difficulties inherent in attempting to regulate CAVM practices, how might a state veterinary board decide whether the "right" acupuncture point or "proper" manual maneuver had been chosen in an animal that failed to respond to or that had been harmed by the application of such treatments?

2. How to Legitimately Prevent Providers of Unproven Practices from Working on Animals

Similarly, it would seem impossible to legitimately try to restrict the practice of alternative veterinary medicine to veterinarians, particularly in light of the fact that no particular scientific or veterinary expertise may be necessary for their application, and that most such modalities are not similarly controlled in human medicine. Indeed, the fact that veterinarians *train* laypeople to apply certain CAVM modalities to animals—and vice versa—makes the claim that individuals who receive or provide such training are somehow unable to apply them without veterinary supervision somewhat specious. Since most people providing alternative therapies to people—be it acupuncture, chiropractic, herbals, or any other modality—are not MDs, by what rationale should it also be assumed that those providing such therapies should be veterinarians? Indeed, there is no rationale for the assertion that veterinarians must necessarily be the only ones who can apply ineffective or palliative therapies. Protests to the contrary from the veterinary profession may be justifiably criticized as turf protection.

3. Should Regulations Be Inclusive?

One argument for regulation of CAVM may be that veterinary medicine should be inclusive and respect the beliefs and practices of a number of practitioners. Indeed, CAVM practitioners, while embracing alternative approaches, routinely endorse scientific approaches to veterinary problems.[27] Should science-minded practitioners be equally open-minded toward CAVM practices?

In a word, "No." The crux of the problem is that science is not and does not strive to be fair or inclusive. In science, all ideas are not treated equally. Only those that have satisfied the test of experiment or can be tested by experiment have any currency. Beautiful ideas, elegant ideas, and even sacrosanct notions from ancient times are not immune from rejection based on experimental data. While science is always open to new ideas, open-mindedness does not mean that all ideas are equal. Meaningful standards of practice can only be established because treatment schemes can be generally developed that are based on the best available evidence of effectiveness.

However, while giving lip service to science, CAVM advocates routinely target science and mainstream veterinary medicine as being inadequate in addressing animal health needs. As such, they actually seem to care very little about inclusiveness, instead attempting to separate their practices from mainstream veterinary practice. Consider this example of a thinly veiled assault on scientific veterinary medical practice: "Picture a car with a low oil warning light. Extinguishing the light will certainly make the sign go away, but will it solve the problem?"[28] This example perpetuates the attack on science that characterizes CAVM and, indeed, alternative medicine in general. The clear implication of such an example is that veterinarians who do not espouse CAVM modalities are so amazingly incompetent that they would "turn out the light" in a manner other than adding oil.

To look at the example in another way, what might someone who addressed the "whole car" do? Wash it, repair the upholstery, and realign the front tires (and at what cost)? Certainly, one would imagine that a good mechanic would attend to needed problems, even troubleshoot for problems that might be expected to be associated with the primary complaint. However, at the same time, one would not be happy with a mechanic who attempted to correct problems that could not be shown to exist with repair techniques that could not be shown to work, particularly if the mechanic charged money for having done so. Nor would one be happy if the mechanic charged for additional services that were not needed or requested. The proper approach to repairing the car is to detect the specific problem (lack of oil), treat it in a targeted fashion (add oil), and make sure that there is no other underlying problem (gasket leak, etc.). There are no other legitimate alternatives to such an approach, either in auto mechanics or in veterinary medicine.

Advocates of CAVM appear to want to be considered as incorporating the best of both worlds. Such an assertion assumes that all competing approaches to veterinary care are somehow equal.† This is certainly not true—the history of medicine is littered with the carcasses of failed therapies. Nevertheless, practitioners of alternative medicine may not be concerned with science or attempts to elucidate the basic scientific mechanism of individual therapies. Knowledge bases in alternative medicine are often derived from clinical observations or personal experience and treatment decisions are generally individualistic and empirical. Indeed, traditional teachings may be passed on in a way that *discourages* questioning and evolution of such practices, instead, encouraging practitioners to rely on their own anecdotal and intuitive experiences as well as those of others.[29]

In addition, therapeutic methods selected from the framework of a social rather than scientific construct soon encounter insoluble paradoxes and irreconcilable contradictions. For example, there are dozens of systems of acupuncture. According to proponents, they all work. There are thousands of other alternative practices, with innumerable variations. How does one rationally decide which ones are most appropriate and which ones to include if not by some objective means? How can one apply a standard of practice when there is none in the applicable field?

Rather than being concerned that regulations be inclusive, regulators should insist that CAVM practitioners attempt to bring their practices into the mainstream via well-established scientific methodology prior to assuming that they are part of veterinary medicine. If particular modalities fail the test of science, the veterinary profession should discard those modalities.

4. Is CAVM Veterinary Medicine?

In considering regulation of CAVM, it is reasonable to consider whether CAVM practices constitute the practice of veterinary medicine. Again, given the paucity of scientific data supporting such practices, particularly in veterinary medicine, the very best that can be said about them is that they are unproven and experimental. However, a number of CAVM practices are essentially disproved, or at least thoroughly discredited, or fly in the face of a large body of evidence (homeopathy, subluxations, energy medicine, therapeutic magnets, mega-vitamin therapy, etc.). As such, the prescription of such practices by professionals would seem to be indefensible, at least from the standpoint of endorsement of them by the veterinary profession.

It is interesting that legal defense of alternative medical or veterinary practices may be mounted with the argument that such practices *do not* constitute

---

†"In many acute situations, treatment may involve aspects of surgery and drug therapy from conventional western technology, along with alternative techniques to provide a complementary whole" (http://www.ahvma.org/; accessed May 5, 2002).

the practice of veterinary medicine. For example, the constitutionality of the Texas regulations was recently challenged in court.[30] The plaintiffs in the Texas suit—a veterinarian who had a homeopathic practice and one of the clients— contended the Texas alternative veterinary medical care regulations were not constitutional because, among other reasons, the practice of homeopathy was different from the practice of "allopathic" medicine[§] and that regulatory veterinary statutes unconstitutionally favored one form of veterinary medicine over another, in violation of the Texas constitution.[31] The suit claimed that the Texas statutes made it seem that homeopathic treatment "somehow involve[s] risks and potential failure greater than the risks and potential failure one might realize from allopathic cures" and that the Texas rules discriminate between various forms of alternative treatment. The veterinarian's client, who was also a plaintiff, claimed that the Texas statutes violated her rights to privacy under the due process clause of the Fourteenth Amendment of the United States Constitution and unfairly limited the client's ability to treat her animal with medications of her own choosing. This case was dismissed after the death of the plaintiff-veterinarian.

Similarly, successful defenses of chiropractic have been mounted on the premise that chiropractic is not medicine and should not be held to the same standards as medicine. Indeed, such arguments have been the foundation of successful defenses mounted on behalf of chiropractors since 1907.[32] For example, in 1998, in Wisconsin, an appellate court ruled that a chiropractor was not liable for the death of a man from lung cancer even though the tumor that killed the man was easily seen on initial radiographs taken by the chiropractor because, unlike physicians, chiropractors are not licensed to diagnose medical problems.** One can easily formulate and anticipate a similar defense

---

§The term *allopathic* medicine is a misnomer. It was coined by the homeopath Samuel Hahnemann to distinguish his practices from competing approaches. The alternative medicine movement uses the term to imply that medicine is unnatural, inflexible, and merely one of many types of medicine from which a consumer can legitimately choose. See Gundling, K. E., When did I become an "allopath"? *Arch Intern Med* 1998; 158(20): 2185–86.

**The chiropractor in question X-rayed the patient and told him that the radiographs indicated that he needed a spinal adjustment. The X ray also showed an abnormal mass near his spine that was missed by the chiropractor, but was later found to be cancer. The patient's family sued the chiropractor for failing to point out the abnormal mass, arguing that doing so would have enabled the patient to obtain earlier diagnosis and treatment, which would have increased his chances of survival. However, the court stated that in Wisconsin chiropractors are limited to treating the spinal column and adjacent tissues, not including the lungs. Whereas the attorney for the family of the deceased argued that if a chiropractor is trained to recognize what is normal on an X ray, he should be able to recognize an abnormality and at least inform a patient about it so medical help can be sought, the chiropractor's attorney and the court disagreed (*NCRHI News* 1998 May/June; 21, #3 http://www.ncahf.org/nl/1998/5-6.html; accessed May 12, 2002).

for the misapplication of chiropractic to animals. Furthermore, the American Veterinary Chiropractic Association has explicitly stated that veterinary chiropractors are not practicing veterinary medicine, and, as such, should not be subjected to regulation by veterinary regulatory boards.

5. The Whole Patient

CAVM approaches challenge veterinary medicine by asserting that they consider the whole patient, and, by implication, that science-based practitioners do not. This is clearly not the case. Good medical practitioners routinely work in a holistic manner. Conversely, CAVM therapists may be narrow in their approach to particular problems, even eschewing proven-effective therapies for therapies from their particular field of interest. In fact, "holism" relates more to the outlook of the practitioner than to the type of medicine that is practiced.

Scientific medicine is far from orthodox, and it is guarded from becoming such by constant testing and change, and by holding to the principle that no idea of the physical world is sacred or immutable. Nor does scientific medicine preclude the arts of compassion and empathy. To the contrary, good veterinary medicine combines both the art and the explicit science of medicine and considers the whole patient in the context of its environment, as well as the client's emotional needs (needs that are not necessarily served by employing costly ineffective therapies). Indeed, the 2001 AVMA Guidelines note that *all* veterinary medicine is "holistic in that it considers all aspects of the animal patient in the context of its environment." Thus, there is no substantive difference between the stated goals of CAVM and that of veterinary medicine in general.

Nevertheless, CAVM practitioners may assert that it is necessary to consider an almost limitless number of factors in deciding which approach or combination of approaches is best suited for the diagnosis and treatment of the patient. However, all of the available evidence suggests that this is not the case. That is, a huge body of research has demonstrated that human judgment cannot compete with a more objective process that involves evaluating a small number of relevant variables, including judgment used in the differential diagnosis and prognosis of medical conditions.[33] When given identical information, statistical procedures are more accurate than are professional judgments. This is even true when professionals are provided additional information that was not used in formulating the statistical procedure. It is also true when professionals are provided with the results of the statistical procedure, in which case professionals identify too many exceptions to the rule[34] and may ignore the statistical evidence.

There is, in fact, no indication that CAVM practices offer any diagnostic or therapeutic advantage over science-based approaches and every reason to believe that no such advantages exist or will be forthcoming, given the long history of their use and concomitant lack of supporting evidence.

6. Can CAVM Be Tested?

CAVM advocates may assert that their methods are so individualized that they cannot be tested by scientific methodology. As such, one could reasonably assert that such practices do not belong in a scientific profession. Nevertheless, such claims would appear to be suspect, in view of the position of the National Institutes of Health that alternative practices are, in fact, amenable to testing.[††]

However, even when tested, many CAVM approaches cannot necessarily be incorporated into a scientific framework. There are hypotheses that simply cannot be accommodated by or reconciled with scientific knowledge. For example, one cannot uncritically accept the proposition that effective remedies can be made by diluting a substance past the point where not a single molecule remains, any more than one can uncritically agree that one's future is foretold by the stars. Indeed, testing of such hypotheses could be reasonably regarded as a waste of time and money, since positive results are unlikely to be obtained, and negative results are unlikely to sway firm beliefs.

7. What Might Be Regulated?

Unfortunately, it is not possible to conduct a meaningful risk/benefit analysis when neither the potential risks nor the potential benefits of a therapy have been fully examined in an objective, scientific way (that is, by the same standards employed to evaluate mainstream therapies). However, it would seem that using an unproven or disproven CAVM therapy in cases where an acceptable and effective treatment already exists or where the patient is at risk for greater suffering if the unproven treatment fails would be unethical[35] and, as such, subject to regulation. For example, an individual veterinarian may think that antibiotics are unnatural or overprescribed; however, in the case of a sick animal, if antibiotics are the most effective treatment, directing someone to an unproven alternative might cause harm and be below the standard of care. Similarly, if an animal is in pain, prescribing an unproven alternative in lieu of a proven-effective therapy runs the risk of causing the animal further suffering. Preventing animal pain, suffering, or distress is one of the moral and ethical foundations for the practice of veterinary medicine, even forming the

---

[††]"Contrary to the assertions of many researchers and alternative practitioners, established methodologies (e.g., experimental trials, observational epidemiology, social survey research) and data-analytic procedures (analysis of variance, logistic regression, multivariate modeling techniques) are quite satisfactory for addressing the majority of study questions related to alternative medicine, from clinical research on therapeutic efficacy to basic science research on mechanisms of pathogenesis and recovery" (Levin, J. S., et al., Quantitative methods in research on complementary and alternative medicine: Methodological manifesto. NIH Office of Alternative Medicine. *Med Care* 1997; 35[11]: 1079–94).

moral and ethical basis for animal euthanasia. Trading a known way of controlling pain for an unproven alternative is morally reprehensible and is a substandard method of care. The well-being of an animal must be kept at the forefront of any consideration of therapy. Regulations should reflect such concerns.

Certainly, existing standards for regulation are applicable to all veterinarians. However, given the lack of information—as well as the false information—about CAVM, it may be difficult for regulators to consider many CAVM practices objectively. Still, in the absence of clear evidence of effectiveness, it may be possible to provide some guidance for some limited regulation of CAVM practices.

1. It is not appropriate to administer a CAVM therapy in lieu of an effective therapy. If such practice occurs, it could be subject to regulatory activity. The level of clinical risk must ultimately be determined.

2. The lack of supporting documentation in a medical record can be used to help demonstrate failure of appropriate care and justify disciplinary action. The evidence supporting the practice would also have to be assessed by the regulators.

3. At the very least, clients must be informed that CAVM practices are experimental. Express, written informed consent should be given to and acknowledged by clients prior to subjecting animals to such treatments, as would be done with any other experimental procedure. Failure to demonstrate such consent could be grounds for regulatory action.

4. Concurrent conventional monitoring and follow-up should be mandatory in the case of any animal treated with any CAVM modality.

5. CAVM therapies may be harmful, at least indirectly, if they necessitate additional expenditures for interventions of unknown benefit.[36] This may also be an area where regulatory action could be considered.

Afterword

The rise of complementary and alternative veterinary medicine (CAVM), as well as alternative medical approaches in human medicine, should provide the animal and human medical community with an occasion to reflect. Scientific medicine must examine where it may have failed to meet what society expects of medical people. For example, more emphasis might be placed in medical education on the importance of empathetic interactions with patients and clients, at the same time that more attention is paid to explaining science as the basis for diagnosis and treatment. Phenomena like CAVM and the accompanying reaction against biotechnology indicate that the public—and all too frequently veterinarians—fails to truly understand biomedical science, and, as a result, fears and distrusts what it does not understand. If public acceptance of science does not keep pace with scientific progress, and acceptance presupposes understanding, a vigorous assault must be launched against scientific illiteracy, combated with the same vigor that has been directed against the inability to read. If it is to be generally embraced, science cannot know and do more and more, while the public comprehends less and less.

CAVM provides a façade of compassion that may be attractive to both consumers and practitioners of veterinary medicine. However, behind this façade, idiosyncratic and unproven approaches are shielded from scientific and skeptical scrutiny. As such, both consumers and providers of such therapies may be drawn to it. Proponents of alternative approaches to veterinary medicine are attempting to gain a larger base for nonscientific, unproven, and disproven practices within the legitimate scientific and veterinary medical frame by political and social, rather than scientific, means. This is worrisome because it threatens to cause direct or indirect harm to animals and clients, as well as to erode the basis by which veterinarians can legitimately claim to have the exclusive right to treat animals.

The veterinary profession has progressed because it adopted a potent methodology to search for scientific truth. That method does not care about the origin of the ideas that it examines. Indeed, practices and hypotheses are welcome to be tested under the auspices of science, which is the essence of open-mindedness. No matter what social and political forces, driven by belief and anecdote, are in current vogue, scientific methodology can be used to decide what should or should not be incorporated into the veterinary therapeutic armamentarium.

Scientific medicine is not simply a social construct and current CAVM practices do not fit into its boundaries. If regulators intend to protect the public and the profession, those regulations must be based on some objective standards. The obvious choice of those standards is science and the best available evidence. Otherwise, the privileged status of the veterinary profession will rely on the legislatively granted imprimatur of professionalism to protect the profession, as well as consumers. However, that imprimatur will be and is being challenged as the profession tacitly endorses unscientific practices that may be equally well applied by nonveterinary professionals (some of whom may even be trained by veterinarians) or even laypeople.

If the requirement for scientific evidence of the effectiveness of medicine were dropped or diminished, and regulations of the practice of veterinary medicine relaxed accordingly, a very possible alternative would be a more democratic approach to medical knowledge and practice. This might begin with weakening of veterinary practice acts. As such, rather than deciding in advance that veterinary medicine must be based in science, and laws and regulations on its practice based accordingly, the marketplace would be allowed to determine what therapies are provided and which prevail. However, under such an approach, veterinary medicine would be reduced to being one more competing approach to medicine. With no favored standard of proof, there can be no legitimately privileged status accorded to practitioners of science-based medicine.

On a social level, in an unregulated free market system, no line could be drawn between validated medicine and quackery. In an "anything goes" approach to medicine, the public could be victimized by unfounded, exaggerated, and false claims, glitzy advertising, anecdote, and nontestable testimonials (which are currently being made by healthcare professionals themselves). Indeed, as regulations regarding standards of proof in the human field have been relaxed, victimization of the public is precisely what has taken place. The 1994 U.S. Dietary Supplement Health and Education Act provides an example of such victimization.[1]

It may be argued that not all of veterinary medicine is science based, so to use such a stringent standard to evaluate nonconforming therapies is inconsistent. If true, the implication is that this might somehow justify the integration of any number of unconventional modalities with a similar dearth of supporting scientific evidence into mainstream medical practice. While this line of reasoning is a logical fallacy (*tu quoque*), at least in human medicine, such an assertion is not accurate.[2] Still, even if scientifically evaluated therapies were the exception rather than the rule in veterinary medicine, it would not be justifiable to abandon science as the standard by which all therapies should be judged and regulated. *Some* standard is necessary by which to regulate the profession, science lays legitimate claim to being the *best* standard, and veterinary medicine lays justifiable claim as the field that relies on science for its knowledge. The profession should insist that all therapies ultimately be judged under the same set of rules.

When veterinarians prescribe and defend unproven alternative therapies, and regulators attempt to regulate them on nonobjective grounds, they are implicitly embracing the free market model for medicine and undercutting the privileged status currently enjoyed by veterinarians. In effect, they are saying and have said that scientific evidence is nothing special. By undercutting scientific authority, those veterinarians are also implying that the socially designated authority that veterinarians have earned over the past decades is arbitrary and has been unjustly granted.

Either veterinarians deserve to be the gatekeepers for animals' health or they do not. If they do, it must be by virtue of something that sets them apart from other would-be animal healers. In the absence of any other viable alternative, that something must be a science-based approach to diagnosis and treatment. If this approach is ignored, veterinarians have no valid claim to being gatekeepers, and they must be prepared to line up and hawk their wares at the market like everyone else. Veterinary medicine is either science based in principle, application, and regulation, or it is not. The profession cannot have it both ways.

Veterinary medicine has come a long way from the turn-of-the-century horse doctors. Only as the standards of veterinary education rose were scientifically trained veterinarians able to distinguish themselves from blacksmiths, empirics, and outright quacks. Current trendy flirtations with unproven and disproven therapeutic modalities jeopardize the hard-won and mutually beneficial marriage between scientific veterinary medicine and society. Valid therapeutic claims and regulation of the profession *must* be made based on objective scientific knowledge, for the good of all involved in the veterinarian-patient-client transaction. If no objective evidence exists to support the safety and efficacy of an alleged therapy, it is not rationally justifiable for a professional to use it under the aegis of a therapeutic alternative, nor can the rights to apply it be protected by statute. If a new therapy is proposed, it must be scientifically tested prior to being generally advocated by the profession. The fact is, therapies that have been scientifically evaluated are more likely to be safe and effective, and their risks better understood, than those that have not been so evaluated.

Clients come to veterinarians with any number of ideas and frames of mind, some of which are radically different from those of the veterinarian. However, scientific medicine can be explained and offered to most clients in a manner that does not conflict with their beliefs. On the other hand, offering magic and unproven modalities—from infinite dilutions to the ever-present but unmeasurable *qi*—is an affront to clients and patients and cheapens the practice of veterinary medicine. If veterinarians truly honor their patients, are they, as a profession, ready to offer them these explanations? Are veterinarians ready to attempt to regulate their profession based on such unscientific traditions?

Speaking to the Medical Society of the District of Columbia in 1913, Dr. John Benjamin Nichols, president of the society, noted words that are as apt today as they were when spoken.

> It may be frankly admitted that there are many short-comings and imperfections in regular medicine. The ranks of the profession contain incompetent and unworthy individuals who at heart are quacks, sectarians and fakers. Low standards of medical education in the past have enabled many inadequately trained persons to obtain the legal right to practice medicine. The most competent practitioners make mistakes. There are limitations to our therapeutic resources, and many conditions in which we are unable to render help, in which, of course, our efficiency is no greater than that of the sectarians. All such objections amount to this: that like other men, we are not perfect and infallible, and our science has not yet attained its complete development. With correct methods and proper motives, scientific medicine alone is in a position to attain the maximum possible of truth and efficiency and the minimum of error and harmfulness.[3]

The mission of veterinary medicine is to elucidate the best path to the prevention and cure of animal diseases and, failing that, to alleviate animal suffering. Veterinarians should not be too particular about using whatever is necessary to help accomplish those goals. However, that does not mean that anything goes. Veterinarians have a professional obligation not only to avoid harm, but also to do some good. They also have the obligation to regulate themselves, so as to help avoid external regulation by people with lesser expertise (among other reasons). The best way to achieve those goals is to rely on scientific methodology, a methodology developed to search for empirical proof.

Even if the boundaries of medicine shift due to social and political forces, empirical methodology can be used to test what should or should not be incorporated into scientific veterinary medicine. It is not logical to ignore this background insofar as application and regulation of unproven or disproven therapies is concerned, nor is it logical to ignore attacks on that background that come from within the profession. Indeed, one might argue the opposite and suggest veterinarians rely on the science-based practice that has made them an admired and respected profession and regulate themselves accordingly. Science has advanced the veterinary profession, as well as protected the interests of veterinary professionals, animals, and clients. It is *the* objective standard by which the profession can regulate itself. If CAVM is indeed an integral part of veterinary medicine, it should be subsumed into the legitimate veterinary medical framework by legitimate and well-established mechanisms. It should not ask for special dispensation.

Appendix

AVMA Guidelines for Complementary and Alternative Veterinary Medicine—2001

INTRODUCTION

These guidelines are intended to help veterinarians make informed and judicious decisions regarding medical approaches known by several terms including "complementary," "alternative," and "integrative." Collectively, these approaches have been described as Complementary and Alternative Veterinary Medicine (CAVM). The AVMA recognizes the interest in and use of these modalities and is open to their consideration.

The AVMA believes that all veterinary medicine, including CAVM, should be held to the same standards. Claims for safety and effectiveness ultimately should be proven by the scientific method. Circumstances commonly require that veterinarians extrapolate information when formulating a course of therapy. Veterinarians should exercise caution in such

These guidelines are reprinted with permission of the AVMA, May 22, 2002.

circumstances. Practices and philosophies that are ineffective or unsafe should be discarded.

TERMINOLOGY

The identification of standard and broadly accepted definitions applicable to CAVM, including the definition of CAVM itself, is challenging. These guidelines identify CAVM as a heterogeneous group of preventive, diagnostic, and therapeutic philosophies and practices. The theoretical bases and techniques of CAVM may diverge from veterinary medicine routinely taught in North American veterinary medical schools or may differ from current scientific knowledge, or both.

It is not the intent of these guidelines to determine or describe the relative value of the individual modalities. The evidence pertaining to, and the practice of, individual CAVM modalities differ. Current examples of CAVM include, but are not limited to, aromatherapy; Bach flower remedy therapy; energy therapy; low-energy photon therapy; magnetic field therapy; orthomolecular therapy; veterinary acupuncture, acutherapy, and acupressure; veterinary homeopathy; veterinary manual or manipulative therapy (similar to osteopathy, chiropractic, or physical medicine and therapy); veterinary nutraceutical therapy; and veterinary phytotherapy.

EDUCATION, TRAINING, AND CERTIFICATION

The AVMA believes veterinarians should ensure that they have the requisite skills and knowledge for any treatment modality they may consider using. The AVMA does not officially recognize diplomate-status or certificates other than those awarded by veterinary specialty organizations that are members of the AVMA American Board of Veterinary Specialties (ABVS), nor has it evaluated the training or education programs of other entities that provide such certificates. Recognition of a veterinary specialty organization by the AVMA requires demonstration of a substantial body of scientific knowledge. The AVMA encourages CAVM organizations to demonstrate such a body of knowledge.

RECOMMENDATIONS FOR PATIENT CARE

The foremost objective in veterinary medicine is patient welfare. Ideally, sound veterinary medicine is effective, safe, proven, and holistic in that it considers all aspects of the animal patient in the context of its environment.

Diagnosis should be based on sound, accepted principles of veterinary medicine. Proven treatment methods should be discussed with the owner or authorized agent when presenting the treatment options available. Informed consent should be obtained prior to initiating any treatment, including CAVM.

Clients usually choose a medical course of action on the advice of their veterinarian. Recommendations for effective and safe care should be based on available scientific knowledge and the medical judgment of the veterinarian.

RESPONSIBILITIES

State statutes define and regulate the practice of veterinary medicine including many aspects of CAVM. These guidelines support the requisite interaction described in the definition of the veterinarian-client-patient relationship.[1] Accordingly, a veterinarian should examine an animal and establish a preliminary diagnosis before any treatment is initiated.

The quality of studies and reports pertaining to CAVM varies; therefore, it is incumbent on a veterinarian to critically evaluate the literature and other sources of information. Veterinarians and organizations providing or promoting CAVM are encouraged to join with the AVMA in advocating sound research necessary to establish proof of safety and efficacy.

Medical records should meet statutory requirements. Information should be clear and complete. Records should contain documentation of client communications and informed consent.

In general, veterinarians should not use treatments that conflict with state or federal regulations. Veterinarians should be aware that animal nutritional supplements and botanicals typically are not subject to premarketing evaluation by the FDA for purity, safety, or efficacy and may contain active pharmacologic agents or unknown substances. Manufacturers of veterinary devices may not be required to obtain premarketing approval by the FDA for assurance of safety or efficacy. Data establishing the efficacy and safety of such products and devices should ultimately be demonstrated. To assure the safety of the food supply, veterinarians should be judicious in the use of products or devices for the treatment of food-producing animals.

If a human health hazard is anticipated in the course of a disease or as a result of therapy, it should be made known to the client.

Notes

Chapter 1

1. Nichols, J. B. Medical sectarianism. *JAMA* 1913; 60(5): 331–37.
2. Mazur, A. Bias in analysis of the laetrile controversy. In *Politics, science and cancer: The laetrile phenomenon,* Markle, E., and Petersen, J., eds. AAAS Selected Symposia. Boulder, CO: Westview Press, 1980; 178.
3. O'Callaghan, F. V., Jordan, N. Postmodern values, attitudes and the use of complementary medicine. *Complement Ther Med* 2003; 11(1): 28–32.
4. Clouser, K., Hufford, D., Morrison, C. What's in a word? *Alt Ther Health Med* 1995; 1(3): 97–98.
5. Gardner, M. *Weird water and fuzzy logic: More notes of a fringe watcher.* Amherst, NY: Prometheus Books, 1996.
6. Randi, J. *The faith healers.* Amherst, NY: Prometheus Books, 1989.
7. Ernst, E. The rise and fall of complementary medicine. *J R Soc Med* 1998; 91(5): 235–36.
8. Watson, R. EU to tighten rules on vitamin pills. *BMJ* 2002; 324: 697
9. Wal-Mart Open Enrollment News. September, 2002.
10. More Medicaid cuts loom for chiropractic (http: //www.chiroweb.com/ archives/21/11/15.html; accessed June 28, 2003).

Chapter 2

1. Kambewa, B. M. D., Mfitilodze, M. W., Hüttner, K., Wollny, C. B. A., et al. The use of indigenous veterinary remedies in Malawi. In *Proceedings of an international conference on ethnoveterinary medicine: Alternatives for livestock development.* Pune, India, 1997.

2. Bartlett, E. *An essay on the philosophy of medical science*. Philadelphia: Lea and Febiger, 1844; 290.

3. Whorton, J. C. *Nature cures: The history of alternative medicine in America*. Oxford: Oxford University Press, 2002; 3–24.

4. Unschuld, P. *Medicine in China: Historical artifacts and images*. Munich: Prestel Verlag, 2000; 7.

5. Unschuld, P. *Chinese medicine*. Brookline, MA: Paradigm Publications, 1998; 3.

6. Kuriyama, S. *Pneuma, qi,* and the problematic of breath. In *The comparison between concepts of life-breath in East and West*, Kawata, Y., Sakai, S., Otsuka, O., eds. Tokyo, Japan: Ishiyaku EuroAmerica, Inc., 1995; 1–32.

7. Unschuld, P. *Medicine in China: A history of pharmaceutics*. Berkeley: University of California Press, 1986.

8. Loewe, M. *Chinese ideas of life and death, faith, myth and reason in the Han period (202 B.C.–A.D. 220)*. London: George Allen and Unwin, Ltd., 1982.

9. Adams, J. N. *Pelagonius and Latin veterinary terminology in the Roman Empire*. Leiden, New York, Köln: E. J. Brill, 1995; 18–34.

10. Unschuld, P. *Medicine in China: A history of ideas*. Berkeley: University of California Press, 1985; 57–58.

11. Epler, D. Bloodletting in early Chinese Medicine and its relation to the origin of acupuncture. *Bull Hist Med* 1980; 54: 357–67.

12. Unschuld, P. Chinese medicine. *Lancet*, 1999; Supp 4: 354.

13. Beyerstein, B., Sampson W. Traditional medicine and pseudoscience in China: A report of the second CSICOP delegation (Part 1). *Skeptical Inquirer*, July/August 1996. See: http://www.cscicop.org

14. Yamada, K. *The origins of acupuncture, moxibustion, and decoction*. Kyoto, Japan: International Research Center for Japanese Studies, 1998; 56.

15. Harper, D. *Early Chinese medical literature: The Mawangdui medical manuscripts*. London: Kegan Paul International, 1997.

16. Mahathero, R. Jivaka and his contribution to medical science. (http://www.mwobd.org/jcms.html; accessed Feb. 6, 2003).

17. Keegan, D. J. *The Huang-Ti Nei-Ching: The structure of the compilation, the significance of the compilation*. Dissertation, 1988. UMI Dissertation Service Order 8916728.

18. Akahori A. The interpretation of classical Chinese medical texts in contemporary Japan: Achievements, approaches, and problems. In *Approaches to traditional Chinese medical literature*, Unschuld, P., ed. Dordrecht: Kluwer Academic Publishers, 1989; 19–27.

19. Prioreschi, P. *A History of medicine*. Volume I1. Omaha, NE: Horatius Press, 1996; 176, 514.

20. Lu, G., Needham, J. *Celestial lancets: A history and rationale of acupuncture and moxa*. Cambridge: Cambridge University Press, 1980; 225–26.

21. Unschuld, P. *Forgotten traditions of ancient Chinese medicine*. Brookline, MA: Paradigm Publications, 1998; 244.
22. Skrbanek, P. Acupuncture: Past, present and future. In *Examining holistic medicine*, Stalker, D., Glymour, C., eds. Buffalo, NY: Prometheus Books, 1985, 182–86.
23. Prioreschi, P. *A History of medicine*, Vol. 1. Omaha, NE: Horatius Press, 1995; 179.
24. Huard, P., Wong, M. *Chinese medicine*. London: Weidenfeld & Nicholson, 1968; 150.
25. Li, Z. *The private life of Chairman Mao: The inside story of the man who made modern China*. London: Chatto & Windus, 1994; 84.
26. *San Jose Mercury News*, July 3, 1998: DD5.
27. *Los Angeles Times*, December 24, 1998: A.
28. Caldwell, J. C. Good health for many: The ESCAP region, 1950–2000. *Asia-Pacific Population Journal* 1999; 14: 4, 21–38.
29. Jackson, P., Morgan, D., eds. *The mission of Friar William of Rubruck*. London: Hakluyt Society (Hakluyt Society, second series, volume 173), 1990; 161–62.
30. Lacassagne, J. Le docteur Louis Berlioz—Introducteur de l'acupuncture en France. *Presse Medicale* 1954; 62: 1359–60.
31. Anon. Acupuncturation. *Medico-Chirugical Review* (London) 1829; 11: 166–67.
32. Cassedy, J. Early uses of acupuncture in the United States, with an addendum (1826) by Franklin Bache, M.D. *Bull. N Y Aca Med* 1974; 50: 8, 892–906.
33. Coxe, E. Observations on asphyxia from drowning. *N Amer Med Surg J* 1826, 292–93.
34. Tavernier, A. *Elements of operative surgery*, Gross, S., trans. and ed. Philadelphia: Grigg, Crissy, Towar & Hogan, Auner, 1829; 55–57.
35. Gross S. *A system of surgery*. Philadelphia: Blanchard & Lea, 1859; 1: 575–76.
36. Bossut, D. Development of veterinary acupuncture in China. *Proc. 16th IVAS Cong Vet Acupunct*. Sept. 13–15, 1990. Noordwijk, Holland: IVAS Sept, 1990; 5.
37. Ramey, D. W., Buell, P. Equine medicine in sixth century China: *Qimin yaoshu*. In *Guardians of the horse II*, Rossdale, P., Green, R., eds. Suffolk, UK: Romney Publications, 2001; 154–61.
38. Sterckx, R. *The animal and the daemon in early China*. State University of New York Press, 2002.
39. *Simu anji ji*, Zhonghua shuju, Beijing, 1957, 29–34
40. Franke, H., von den Dreisch, A. Zur traditionellen Kamelheilkunde in China. *Sudhoffs Archiv* 1997; 81 (1): 84–89.

41. Xu, Changle, ed. *Xinke zhushi ma niu to jing da quanji* [*Newly printed anno-tated great collection of equine, ox, and camel classics*]. Beijing: Nongye chu-pansha, 1988.

42. *Ryoyaku baryo benkai* [*Explanations of good medicinals for treating horses*], Yedo, 1859 (org. 1759), 2, 24B.

43. Kao, F. F., Kao, J. J. Veterinary acupuncture. *Am J Chin Med* 1974; 2(1): 89–102.

44. Jochle. W. Veterinary acupuncture in Europe and America: Past and present. *Am J Acupuncture* 1978; 6(2): 149–56.

45. Schoen, A., ed. *Veterinary acupuncture: Ancient art to modern medicine.* St. Louis: Mosby, 1994; 315; Klide, A., Kung, S., *Veterinary acupuncture.* University of Pennsylvania Press, 1977; 265–70.

46. Nogier P. F. M. Le pavillion de l'Orielle. *Bull Societe l'Acupuncture* 1957; 25: 25.

47. Hsu E. Innovations in acumoxa: Acupuncture analgesia, scalp and ear acupuncture in the People's Republic of China. *Soc Sci Med* 1996; 42(3): 421–30.

48. Nishimura, N. [Anesthesiology in People's Republic of China in the year 2001]. Masui 2002 Mar; 51(3): 314–17 [in Japanese].

49. Soulié de Morant, G. *Chinese acupuncture*, English edition edited by Zmiewski, P. Brookline, MA: Paradigm Publications, 1994.

50. White, S., in *Veterinary acupuncture: Ancient art to modern medicine*, ed. Schoen, A. St. Louis, MO: Mosby, 1994; 584.

51. Panzer, R. A comparison of the traditional Chinese versus transposition-al zangfu organ association acupoint locations in the horse. *Am J Chin Med* 1993; 21(2): 119–31.

52. Despeux, C., Apercu historique de l'art veterinaire en Chine. *Revue d'acuponcture veterinaire* 1981; 9: 21–22.

53. *The principles and practical use of acupuncture anesthesia*. Hong Kong: Medicine and Health Publishing, 1974.

54. Heerde, M. Pferdeklassiker. *Needling: Manner and method*; PhD Thesis, 1998; 33–34.

55. Heerde, M. Pferdeklassiker. *Song on the observation of the hair whorls of good and bad horses*; PhD Thesis, 1998; 33–34.

56. Schoen, A., ed. *Veterinary acupuncture: Ancient art to modern medicine.* St. Louis, MO: Mosby, 1994; 14.

57. Guo HuaiXi: Xinke zhushi ma niu to jing da quan ji [Newly printed and annotated horse, ox, and camel classics], Nongye chuban she, Beijing, 1988 (org. 1795); 107–9.

58. White S. Acupuncture of horses in China. In *Veterinary acupuncture: Ancient art to modern medicine*, Schoen, A., ed. St. Louis, MO: Mosby, 1994; 581.

59. Altman S. Small animal acupuncture: Scientific basis and clinical applications. In *Complementary and alternative veterinary medicine: Principles and practice*, Schoen, A., Wynn, S., eds. St. Louis, MO: Mosby, 1998; 154.

60. Chinese Rotunda at the University of Pennsylvania Museum of Archaeology and Anthropology (http://www.upenn.edu/museum/Collections/china.html; accessed April 16, 2003).

61. Epler, D. Bloodletting in early Chinese medicine and its relation to the origin of acupuncture. *Bull Hist Med* 1980; 54: 357–67.

62. Paris, S. V. A history of manipulative therapy through the ages and up to the current controversy in the United States. *J Man and Manip Therapy* 2000; 8(2): 66–77.

63. Keating, J. *BJ of Davenport: The early years of chiropractic*. Association for the History of Chiropractic, Davenport, IA, 1997.

64. Palmer, D. D. *The chiropractor's adjuster, or the text-book of the science, art and philosophy of chiropractic*. Portland, OR: Portland Printing House Company, 1910; 17–19.

65. Leach, R. A. *The chiropractic theories*. 3d ed. Baltimore: Williams & Wilkins, 1994; 359.

66. United States District Court for the Northern District of Illinois, Eastern Division. *Chester A. Wilk, et al., Plaintiffs, v. American Medical Association, et al., Defendants*, No. 76 C 3777, 25, Sept., 1987.

67. Nelson, C. F. The subluxation question. *Journal of Chiropractic Humanities* 1997; 7: 46–55.

68. Splaude, T. C. Chiropractic for horses. *Fountain Head News*, 1921; 10(47): 1.

69. *Fountain Head News*. Palmer School of Chiropractic, Davenport, IA, 1923.

70. Palmer, B. J. *It's as simple as that*. Palmer College of Chiropractic, Davenport, IA, 1944; 33, 35–36.

71. Galinas, M. A chiropractic approach to veterinary problems. *Digest of Chiropractic Economics* 1980; 22(4): 41–42.

72. Myles, A. Veterinary chiropractic. . . feasible, practical and proves chiropractic premise. *Digest of Chiropractic Economics* 1980; 23(3): 17–19, 109, 111, 113–14 (Part One); 1980; 23(4): 58, 60, 62, 65–66 (Part Two).

73. Smithcors, J. F. *The American veterinary profession: Its background and development*. Ames: Iowa State University Press, 1963; 554.

74. Chandler, G. H. Talking of adjustments. Am J Clin Med 1923 Apr: 283–87.

75. Taylor, L. L., Romano, L. Veterinary chiropractic. *Can Vet J* 1999 Oct; 40(10): 732–35.

76. Willoughby, S. Chiropractic care. In *Complementary and alternative veterinary medicine*, Schoen, A., Wynn, S., eds. St. Louis, MO: Mosby, 1998; 185–200.

77. Haussler, K. K. Back problems: Chiropractic evaluation and management. *Vet Clin North Am Equine Pract* 1999 Apr; 15(1): 195–209.
78. Hahnemann, S. *Organon of homoeopathic medicine,* 3d American ed. New York: William Raddle, 1849; 29, 31, 38.
79. King, L. S. *The medical world of the eighteenth century.* Chicago: University of Chicago Press, 1958; 159–62.
80. Raso, J. *The expanded dictionary of metaphysical healthcare: Alternative medicine, paranormal healing and related methods.* The Georgia Council Against Health Fraud, 1998; 136.
81. Hahnemann, S. *Organon of homoeopathic medicine,* op. cit.
82. Haehl, R. *Samuel Hahnemann—His life and work.* Jain Publishers, 1971.
83. Hahnemann, S. *The chronic diseases.* New York, 1846; 141.
84. Park, R. L. *Voodoo science: The road from foolishness to fraud.* Oxford: Oxford University Press, 2000.
85. http://www.digibio.com; accessed June 28, 2003.
86. Ransom, S. *Homoeopathy: What are we swallowing?* East Sussex, England: Credence Pub., 1999.
87. Hahnemann, S. *Materia medica pura.* Charles Hempel, trans. New York: Raddle, 1846.
88. Wagner, M. Is homeopathy "new science" or "new age?" *Sci Rev Alt Med* 1997; 1(1): 7–12.
89. Holmes, O. W. *Homeopathy and its kindred delusions.* Boston, 1842.
90. Whorton, J. C. *Nature cures: The history of alternative medicine in America.* Oxford, England: Oxford University Press, 2002; 70.
91. Hering, C., in Hahnemann, S., *Organon of homoeopathic medicine,* Preface to the first American Edition, 1849.
92. Rothstein, W. G. *American physicians in the nineteenth century: From sects to science.* Reprint edition. Baltimore, MD: Johns Hopkins University Press, 1992; 164, 239–41.
93. Hahnemann, S. *Materia,* vol. 2, op. cit., 763–64.
94. Ernst, E. "Neue Deutsche Heilkunde": Complementary/Alternative medicine in the Third Reich. *Comp Ther Med* 2001; 9(1): 49–51.
95. Kaufman, M. *Homeopathy in America: The rise and fall of a medical heresy.* Baltimore, MD: Johns Hopkins Press, 1971.
96. Fye, W. B. Nitroglycerin: A homeopathic remedy. *Circulation* 1986; 73: 21–29.
97. Haller, J. S. Aconite: A case study in doctrinal conflict and the meaning of scientific medicine. *Bull NY Acad Med* 1984; 60: 888–904.
98. Nicholls, P. A. *Homeopathy and the medical profession.* London: Croom Helm, 1998.
99. Ernst, E. Homeopathy revisited. *Arch Intern Med* 1996; 156: 2162–64.

100. Day, C. *Homoeopathic treatment of small animals; Principles and practice.* London: C.W. Daniels, 1992.
101. Hass, K. B. Animal therapy over the ages. *Veterinary Heritage,* 1999; 22(2): 39–40.
102. Smithcors, J. F. *Evolution of the veterinary art: A narrative account to 1850.* Kansas City, MO: Veterinary Medicine Publishing Company, 1957; 373–75.
103. Schaeffer J.C., *New manual of homoeopathic veterinary medicine.* New York: William Radde, 1863; xv.
104. Schaeffer, op. cit., xi.
105. Pitcairn, R. Hahnemann's discovery of psora and its significance in the treatment of animals. *J Am Holistic Vet Med Assoc* 1996; 15: 20–21.
106. Dun, F. *Veterinary medicines: Their actions and uses.* Toronto, Canada: JA Carveth & Co., 1904.
107. Kaufman, M. *Homeopathy in America—the rise and fall of a medical heresy.* Baltimore, MD: Johns Hopkins University, 1971.
108. Kleiner, S. M. The true nature of herbs. *Phys Sports Med* 1995; 23: 13–14.
109. Akerele, O. Nature's medicinal bounty: Don't throw it away. *World Health Forum* 1993; 14: 390–95.
110. Duran-Reynals, M. L. *The fever-bark tree.* Garden City, NY: Doubleday, 1946.
111. Blanton, W. P. *Medicine in Virginia in the seventeenth century.* Richmond, VA: William Byrd Press, 1930.
112. Haller, J. S., Jr. *Kindly medicine.* Kent, OH: Kent State University Press, 1997.
113. Kleiner, op. cit.
114. Ackernecht, E. H. The American Medical Association and the cultivation of the cinchona tree in the United States. *JAMA* 1943; 123: 375.
115. Huxtable, R. Safety of botanicals: Historical perspective. *Proc West Pharmacol Soc* 1998; 41: 1–10.
116. Osol, A., Farrar G. E., eds. *The dispensatory of the United States of America.* 25th ed. Philadelphia, PA: J.B. Lippincott, 1955: 444–60.
117. Eisenberg, D. M., Kaptchuk, T. J. The herbal history of digitalis: Lessons for alternative medicine (Response). *JAMA* 2000; 283: 884.
118. Huxtable, op. cit.
119. Angell, M., Kassirer, J. P. Alternative medicine—the risks of untested and unregulated remedies. *N Engl J Med* 1998; 339: 839–41.
120. Huxtable, op. cit.
121. Haas, K. B. Animal therapy over the ages: 4. Early botanical medicine. *Veterinary Heritage* 2000; 23(1): 6–8.

122. Vogel, V. J. *American Indian medicine*. Norman: University of Oklahoma Press, 1970.
123. Merillat, L. A., Campbell, D. M. *Veterinary military history of the United States*. Kansas City, MO: Haver-Glover Laboratories, 1935.
124. Hiscox, G. D., Sloane, T. O., Eisensen, H. E., eds. *Fortunes in formulas for home, farm and workshop*. New York: Books, Inc., 1957.
125. Wulff-Tilford, M. L., Tilford, G. *Herbs for pets*. Bowtie Press, 1999.
126. Mourino, M. R. From Thales to Lauterbur, or from the lodestone to MR imaging: Magnetism and medicine. *Radiology* 1991; 180: 593–612.
127. Licht, S. *History of electrotherapy: Therapeutic electricity and ultraviolet radiation*. 2d ed. New Haven, CT: Elizabeth Licht; 1967: 1–70.
128. Kane, K., Taub, A. A history of local electrical analgesia. *Pain* 1975; 1: 125–38.
129. Kellaway, P. The part played by electric fish in the early history of bio-electricity and electrotherapy. *Bull Hist Med* 1946; 20: 112–37.
130. Peregrinus, P. *Epistola Petri Peregrini de Maricourt ad Sygerum de Foucaucourt, Militem, De Magnete*. Italy: Privately published; 1289.
131. Morgagni, J. B. *De Sedibas exercise test causis morborum per anatomen indigatis*. Italy: Privately published; 1761.
132. Quinan, J. R. The use of the magnet in medicine. *Maryland Med J* 1885; 14: 460–65.
133. Macklis, R. M. Magnetic healing, quackery, and the debate about the health effects of electromagnetic fields. *Ann Intern Med* 1993; 118: 376–83.
134. Butterfield, J. Dr. Gilbert's magnetism. *Lancet* 1991; 338: 1576–79.
135. *Catalogue of the Scientific Community* (http://es.rice.edu/ES/humsoc/ Galileo/Catalog/Files/guericke.html; accessed March 5, 2003).
136. Hauksbee, F. *Biography—Catalog of the scientific community* (Francis Hauksbee) Compiled by Richard S. Westfall, Dept of History and Philosophy of Science, Indiana University: (http://es.rice.edu/ES/ humsoc/Galileo/Catalog/Files/hauksbee.html).
137. Watson, W. The electrical boy (http://search.excite.com/search.gw? search=Francis+Hauksbee&sorig=netscape; 1748).
138. Colwell, H. A. An essay on the history of electrotherapy and diagnosis. London: Heinemann, 1922.
139. Cavendish, H. An account of some attempts to imitate the effects of the Torpedo fish by electricity. *Phil Trans B* 1776; 66: 196–225.
140. Hackman, W. D. Researches of Dr. Van Marum (1750–1837) on the influence of electricity on animals and plants. *Med Hist* 1972; 16: 11–26.
141. Mesmer F. A. *Memoire sur la decouverte du magnetisme animal*. Geneva. 1779.

142. Mesmer, F. A. G. B. (trans.). *Mesmerism* (translation of the original writings of F. A. Mesmer). Los Altos, CA: Kauffman, 1980.

143. Mackay, C. *Extraordinary popular delusions and the madness of crowds.* London. 1852.

144. Franklin, B. *Report of the commission charged by the king of France with the examination of animal magnetism.* Paris: Bailly, 1784.

145. Young, J. H. *The toadstool millionaires.* Princeton: Princeton University Press, 1961; 17–30.

146. Faraday, M. On volta-electric induction, and the evolution of electricity from magnetism. *Lancet* 1831–32; 2: 246–48.

147. Francis, J. B. Extracting teeth by galvanism. *Dent Rep* 1858; 1: 65–69.

148. McQuillen, J. H., Flagg, J. F., Buckingham, T. L., et al. Galvanism in extracting teeth. *Dent Rep* 1859; 1: 113–15.

149. Oliver, W. G. *Electrical anaesthesia, comprising a brief history of its discovery, a synopsis of experiments, also full directions for its application in surgical and dental operations.* Buffalo, NY: Murray, Rockwell and Co., 1858.

150. Althaus, J. *A treatise on medical electricity, theoretical and practical, and its use in the treatment of paralysis, neuralgia and other diseases.* London: Trubner, 1859.

151. Holbrook, S. H. *The golden age of quackery.* New York: Macmillan, 1959; 18–32.

152. Peterson, F., Kennelly, A. E. Physiological experiments with magnets at the Edison laboratory. *NY Med J* 1892; 56: 729–32.

153. Gwathmey, J. T. *Anesthesiology.* New York: Appleton and Company, 1914; 628–43.

154. Shaw, R. C. Variations in the sensibility to pressure pain caused by nerve stimulation in man. *J Physiol* (London) 1924; 58: 288–93.

155. Milstead, K. L., Davis, J. B., Dobelle, M. Quackery in the medical device field. *Proceedings of the Second National AMA/FDA Congress on Medical Quackery.* Washington, DC; 1963.

156. Brennan, B. A. *Hands of light: A guide to healing through the human energy field.* New York: Bantam Age Books, 1988.

157. Wheeler, L. R. *Vitalism: Its history and validity.* London: Witherby, 1930.

158. Goldberg, B. Heliotherapy. *Arch Phys Ther* 1930; 11: 263.

159. Needham, J., Weit-Djen, L. *Science and civilisation in China.* New York: Cambridge University Press, 1983; vol 5, pt 5, 181–84.

160. Downes, A., Blunt, T. P. Researches on the effect of light upon bacteria and other organisms. *Proc Roy Soc London* 1877; 26: 488.

161. Finsen, N. R. Remarks on the red-light treatment of smallpox. *Br Med J* 1903; 1: 1297.

162. Pleasonton, A. J. *The influence of the blue ray of sunlight and the blue colour of the sky in developing health in developing animal and vegetable life, in arresting*

disease, and in restoring health in acute and chronic disorders to human and domestic animals. Philadelphia: Claxton, Remsen and Haffelfinger, 1876.

163. Kellogg, J. H. *Light therapeutics*. Battle Creek, MI: Modern Medicine Publishing, 1927.

164. Spectro-chrome therapy. *JAMA* 1924; 83: 321.

165. http://www.bioscanlight.com/; accessed March 5, 2003.

166. Licht, S. *History of ultraviolet therapy in therapeutic electricity and ultraviolet radiation*. 2d ed. New Haven CT: Elizabeth Licht, 1967; 191–212.

167. Mester, E., et al. Effect of laser rays on wound healing. *Am J Surg* 1971; 122: 532.

168. Mester, E., Mester, A. F., Mester, A. The biomedical effects of laser application. *Lasers Surg Med* 1985; 5: 31.

169. http://www.fda.gov/cdrh/manual/510kprt1.html; accessed July 12, 2003.

170. Hansern, H. J., Thoroe, U. Low power laser biostimulation of chronic oro-facial pain: A double-blind placebo controlled cross-over study in 40 patients. *Pain* 1990; 43: 169–79.

Chapter 3

1. Rollin, B. E. *The Frankenstein syndrome: Ethical and social issues in the genetic engineering of animals*. New York: Cambridge University Press, 1995.

2. Rollin, B. E. *The unheeded cry: Animal consciousness, animal pain and science, expanded edition*. Ames: Iowa State University Press, 1998.

3. Crick, F. *Of molecules and men*. Seattle: University of Washington Press, 1966.

4. Flexner, A. Medical education in the United States and Canada: A report to the Carnegie Foundation for the Advancement of Teaching. Bulletin Number Four. New York, 1910.

5. Ober, K. P. The Pre-Flexnerian reports: Mark Twain's criticism of medicine in the United States. *Annals of Internal Medicine* 1997 Jan 15; 126: 157–63.

6. Sacks, O. W. *Awakenings*. New York: Harper Perennial, 1990.

7. McMillan, F. Comfort as the primary goal in veterinary medical practice. *JAVMA* 1998; 212(9): 1370–74.

8. McMillan, F. Influence of mental states on somatic health in animals. *JAVMA* 1999; 214(8): 1221–25.

9. McMillan, F. Effects of human contact on animal well-being. *JAVMA* 1999; 215(11): 1592–98.

10. McMillan, F. Quality of life in animals. *JAVMA* 2000; 216(12): 1904–10.

11. Callahan, D. Death and the research imperative. *NEJM* 2000; 342(9): 654–56.

12. Rollin, B. E. The right to die. In *Principles of thanatology*, Kutcher, A., Carr, A., eds. New York: Columbia University Press, 1987.

13. Ferrel, B. R., Rhiner, M. High-tech comfort—ethical issues in cancer pain management for the 1990s. *Journal of Clinical Ethics* 1991; 2, 108–15.
14. Rollin, B. E. Some conceptual and ethical concerns about current views of pain. *Pain Forum* 1999; 8(2): 78–83.
15. Dohoo, S. E., Dohoo, I. R. Factors influencing the postoperative use of analgesics in dogs and cats by Canadian veterinarians. *Can Vet J* 1996; 36: 552–56.
16. Kitchell, R., Guinan, M. The nature of pain in animals. In *The experimental animal in biomedical research*, vol. I, Rollin, B., Kesel, M., eds. Boca Raton: CRC Press, 1989.
17. Levin, J. S., et al. Quantitative methods in research on complementary and alternative medicine. A methodological manifesto. NIH Office of Alternative Medicine. *Med Care* 1997; 35(11): 1079–94.
18. Imrie, R., Ramey, D. W. The evidence for evidence-based medicine. *Complement Ther Med* 2000; 8(2): 123–26.

Chapter 4

1. See especially B. E. Rollin, *Veterinary medical ethics: Theory and cases* (Ames: Iowa: Iowa State University Press, 1999).
2. Rosenthal, D. *Experimental effects in behavioral research*. New York: Appleton, 1966.
3. Committee on Children with Disabilities. American Academy of Pediatrics: Counseling families who choose complementary and alternative medicine for their child with chronic illness of disability. *Pediatrics* 2001; 107(3): 598–601.
4. *Pediatrics*, op. cit.
5. Siegler, M., Osmond, H. *Models of madness, models of medicine*. New York: Harper Colophon, 1974.
6. Rollin, B. E. The use and abuse of Aesculapian authority in veterinary medicine. *J Am Vet Med Assoc* 2002; 220(8): 1144–49.
7. Ramey, D., Rollin, B. E. Ethical aspects of proof and alternative therapies. *J Am Vet Med Assoc* 2001; 218(3): 343–46.
8. McMillan, F. The placebo effect in veterinary medicine. *J Am Vet Med Assoc* 1999; 215(7): 992–98.
9. Hrobjartsson, A., and Gotzsche, T. C. Is the placebo powerless? An analysis of clinical trials comparing placebo with no treatment. *NEJM* 2001; 344(21): 1594–1602.

Chapter 5

1. Motherby, G. *New medical dictionary*. 2d ed. London, 1785.
2. Pepper, O. H. P. A note on the placebo. *Am J Pharmacy* 1945; 117: 409–12.
3. *Dorland's illustrated medical dictionary*. 29th ed. Philadelphia, PA: W.B. Saunders Company, 2000: 1393.

4. Grunbaum, A. The placebo concept in medicine and psychiatry. *Psychol Med* 1986; 16(1): 19–38.

5. For example, see A. K. Shapiro and E. Shapiro, *The powerful placebo: From ancient priest to modern physician* (Baltimore, MD: Johns Hopkins University Press, 1997).

6. Moerman, D. E. General medical effectiveness and human biology: Placebo effects in the treatment of ulcer disease. *Med Anthropol Quart* 1983; 14: 3–16.

7. Kienle, G. S., Kiene, H. The powerful placebo effect; fact or fiction. *J Clin Epidemiol* 1997; 50(12): 1311–18.

8. Hrobjartsson, A., Gotzsche, T. C. Is the placebo powerless? An analysis of clinical trials comparing placebo with no treatment. *NEJM* 2001; 344(21): 1594–1602.

9. Walker, R. D. Antimicrobial chemotherapy. In *Current therapy in equine medicine*, III, Robinson, N. E., ed. Philadelphia, PA: W.B. Saunders Co., 1992.

10. Schwarz, R., Heim, M. Psychosocial considerations about spontaneous remission of cancer. *Onkologie* 2000, Oct; 23(5): 432–35.

11. Whitney, C. W., Von Korff, M. Regression to the mean in treated versus untreated chronic pain. *Pain* 1992; 50(3): 281–85.

12. Wickström, G., Bendix, T. The "Hawthorne effect"—What did the original Hawthorne studies actually show? *Scand J Environ Health* 2000; 26(4): 363–67.

13. James, S. Was there a Hawthorne effect? *Am J Sociol* 1992; 98: 451–68.

14. Freemantle, N., Henry, D., Maynard, A., et al. Promoting cost-effective prescribing. *BMJ* 1995; 310: 955–56.

15. Pavlov, I. P. *Conditioned reflexes*. London: Oxford Press, 1927; 23–78.

16. Voudouris, N. J., Peck, C. L., Coleman, G. Conditioned placebo responses. *J Pers Soc Psychol* 1985; 48: 47–53.

17. ter Riet, G., et al. Is placebo analgesia mediated by endogenous opioids? A systematic review. *Pain* 1998 Jun; 76(3): 273–75.

18. Brody, H. The placebo response: Recent research and implications for family medicine. *J Fam Pract* 2000; 49(7): 649–54.

19. Kaptchuk, T. J. The placebo effect in alternative medicine: Can the performance of a healing ritual have clinical significance? *Ann Intern Med* 2002; 136(11): 817–25.

20. Katptchuk, T. J., Eisenberg, D. M. The persuasive appeal of alternative medicine. *Ann Intern Med* 1998; 129: 1061–65.

21. Thomas, K. B. General practice consultations: Is there any point in being positive? *Br Med J (Clin Res Ed)* 1987; 294: 1200–2.

22. Adler, H. M., Hammett, V. B. The doctor-patient relationship revisited. An analysis of the placebo effect. *Ann Intern Med* 1973; 78: 595–98.

23. Csordas, T. J. The rhetoric of transformation in ritual healing. *Cult Med Psych* 1983; 7: 333–75.
24. Kirmeyer, I. J. Improvisation and authority in illness meaning. *Cult Med Psych* 1994; 18: 183–214.
25. McMillan, F. D. The placebo effect in animals. *J Am Vet Med Assoc* 1999; 215(7): 1999.
26. Gantt, W. H., et al. Effect of person. *Conditional Reflex* 1966; 1: 18–35.
27. Lynch, B. Heart rate changes in the horse to human contact. *Psychophysiology* 1974; 11: 472–78.
28. Newton, J. F., Ehrlich, W. W. Coronary blood flow in dogs: Effect of person. *Conditional Reflex* 1966; 1: 81.
29. Gross, W. B. The benefits of tender loving care. *Int J Stud Anim Prob* 1980; 1: 147–49.
30. Heinsworth, P. H., Brand, A., Willems, P. J. The behavioral response of sows to the presence of human beings and their productivity. *Livestock Prod Sci* 1981; 8: 67–74.
31. Bok, S. The ethics of giving placebos. *Sci Am* 1974; 231: 17–23.
32. Weihrauch, T. R., Gauler, T. C. Placebo—efficacy and adverse effects in controlled clinical trials. *Arzneimittelforschung* 1999 May; 49(5): 385–93.
33. Gillon, R. Medical ethics: Four principles plus attention to scope. *BMJ* 1994; 309: 184–88.
34. Katz, J. The silent world of doctor and patient. New York: The Free Press, 1984; 189–95.

Chapter 6

1. Thomas, K. B. General practice consultation; Is there a point in being positive? *BMJ Clin Res Ed* 1987; 294: 1200–1202.
2. Burstein, H. Discussing complementary therapies with cancer patients: What should we be talking about? *J Clin Oncol* 2000; 18: 2501–4.
3. Holland, J. C. Use of alternative medicine—a marker for distress? *NEJM* 1999; 340: 1758–59.
4. Burstein, H., et al. Use of alternative medicine by women with early-stage breast cancer. *NEJM* 1999; 340: 1733–39.
5. Paltiel, O., et al. Determinants of the use of complementary therapies by patients with cancer. *J Clin Oncol* 2001; 12: 468–71.
6. Sollner, W., et al. Use of complementary and alternative medicine by cancer patients is not associated with perceived distress or poor compliance with standard treatment but with active coping behavior: A survey. *Cancer* 2000; 89: 873–80.
7. Ramos-Remus, C., et al. Assessment of health locus of control in the use of nonconventional remedies by patients with rheumatic disease. *J Rheumatol* 1999; 26: 2468–74.

8. Wortman, C. B. Some determinants of perceived control. *J Personality & Soc Psych* 1975; 31: 282–94.

9. Thompson, S. C., et al. Maintaining perceptions of control: Finding perceived control in low-control circumstances. *J Personality & Soc Psych* 1993; 64: 293–304.

10. Howard, K. I., et al. The dose-response relationship in psychotherapy. *Am Psych* 1986; 41: 159–64.

11. Impellizeri, J. A., Tetrick, M. A., Muir, P. Effect of weight reduction on clinical signs of lameness in dogs with hip osteoarthritis. *J Am Vet Med Assoc* 2000 Apr 1; 216(7):1089–91.

12. Polivy, J., Herman, C. P. The effects of resolving to diet on restrained and unrestrained eaters: The "false hope syndrome." *Int J Eat Disord* 1999 Dec; 26(4): 434–47.

13. Beyerstein, B. L. Social and judgmental biases that make inert treatments seem to work. *Sci Rev Alt Med* 1999; 3(2): 20–33.

14. Baumeister, R. F., Heatherton, T. F., Tice, D. M. When ego threats lead to self-regulation failure: Negative consequences of high self-esteem. *J Personality and Soc Psych* 1993; 64: 141–56.

15. Festinger, L. *A theory of cognitive dissonance.* Stanford, CA: Stanford University Press, 1957.

Chapter 7

1. Lynöe, N. Ethical and professional aspects of the practice of alternative medicine. *Scan J Soc Med* 1992; 20(4): 217–25.

2. Rothstein, W. G. *American physicians in the nineteenth century: From sects to science.* Baltimore: Johns Hopkins Press, 1972.

3. Starr, P. *The social transformation of American medicine.* New York: Basic Books, 1982.

4. Daubert v. Merrell Dow Pharmaceuticals, Inc., 509 U.S. 579 (1993); *Kumho Tire Co. v. Carmichael,* 119 S.Ct. 1167 (1999).

5. Hoffer, L. J. Complementary or alternative medicine: The need for plausibility. *CMAJ* 2003; 168(2): 180–82.

6. Ernst, E. Complementary medicine—scrutinizing the alternatives. *Lancet* 1993; 341: 1626.

7. Feinstein, A. R., Horwitz, R. I. Problems in the "evidence" of "evidence-based medicine." *Am J Med* 1997; 103(6): 529–35.

8. Krumholz, H. M., et al. Aspirin for secondary prevention after acute myocardial infarction in the elderly: prescribed use and outcomes. *Ann Intern Med* 1996; 124(3): 292–8.

9. Krumholz, H. M., et al. National use and effectiveness of beta-blockers for the treatment of elderly patients after acute myocardial infarction: National Cooperative Cardiovascular Project. *JAMA* 1998; 280(7): 623–9.

10. Mitchell, J. B., et al. What role do neurologists play in determining the costs and outcomes of stroke patients? *Stroke* 1996; 27(11): 1937–43.
11. Wong, J. H., Findlay, J. M., Suarez-Almazor, M. E. Regional performance of carotid endarterectomy. Appropriateness, outcomes, and risk factors for complications. *Stroke* 1997; 28(5): 891–8.
12. Kellett, J., Clarke, J. Comparison of "accelerated" tissue plasminogen activator with streptokinase for treatment of suspected myocardial infarction. *Med Decis Making* 1995; 15(4): 297–310.
13. Turpin, R. Characterization of quack theories (http: //www.chewable. com/hypatian/quack.htm).
14. Moroz, A. Issues in acupuncture research: The failure of quantitative methodologies and the possibilities for viable, alternative solutions. *Am J Acupunct* 1999; 27(1–2): 95–103
15. Elorriaga, C. A., Hanna, S. E., Fargas-Babjak, A. Reporting of clinical details in randomized controlled trials of acupuncture for the treatment of migraine/headaches and nausea/vomiting. *J Altern Complement Med* 2003; 9(1): 151–59.
16. Kalauokalani, D., Sherman, K. J., Cherkin, D. C. Acupuncture for chronic low back pain: Diagnosis and treatment patterns among acupuncturists evaluating the same patient. *South Med J.* 2001; 94(5): 486–92.
17. Rabinstein, A. A., Shulman, L. M. Acupuncture in clinical neurology. *Neurolog* 2003; (3): 137–48.
18. Acupuncture: Searching for benefits. *Prescrire Int* 2001 Jun; 10(53): 84–88.
19. Ramey, D. W., Sampson, W. Review of the evidence for the clinical efficacy of human acupuncture. *Sci Rev Alt Med* 2001; 5(4): 195–201.
20. Mayer, D. J. Acupuncture: An evidence-based review of the clinical literature. *Annu Rev Med* 2000; 51: 49–63.
21. Nishimura, N. [Anesthesiology in People's Republic of China in the year 2001] *Masui* 2002; 51(3): 314–17.
22. His-chen, K., Nai-huang, T. *Wen-hui pao*, October 22, 1980. In *Medicine in China: A history of ideas*, Unschuld, P. Berkeley: University of California Press, 1985; 361–66.
23. Scott, S. Developments in veterinary acupuncture. *Acupunct Med* 2001; 19(1): 27–31.
24. Gaynor, J. S. Acupuncture for management of pain. *Vet Clin North Am Small Anim Pract* 2000; 30(4): 875–84
25. Hielm-Bjorkman, A., et al. Double-blind evaluation of implants of gold wire at acupuncture points in the dog as a treatment for osteoarthritis induced by hip dysplasia. *Vet Rec* 2001; 149(15): 452–56.
26. Merritt, A. M., et al. Evaluation of a method to experimentally induce colic in horses and the effects of acupuncture applied at the Guan-yuan-shu (similar to BL-21) acupoint. *Am J Vet Res* 2002; 63(7): 1006–11.

27. Parent, J. M. Clinical management of canine seizures. *Vet Clin North Am Small Anim Pract* 1988; 18(4): 947–64.
28. Kloster, R., et al. The effect of acupuncture in chronic intractable epilepsy. *Seizure* 1999; 8(3): 170–74.
29. Stavem, K., et al. Acupuncture in intractable epilepsy: Lack of effect on health-related quality of life. *Seizure* 2000; 9(6): 422–26.
30. Carlsson, C. Acupuncture mechanisms for clinically relevant long-term effects—reconsideration and a hypothesis. *Acupunct Med* 2002; 20(2–3): 82–99.
31. Ramey, D. W., Lee, M. L., Messer, N. T. A review of the Western language equine acupuncture literature. *J Eq Vet Sci* 2001; 21(2): 56–60.
32. Linde, K., et al. The methodological quality of randomized controlled trials of homeopathy, herbal medicines and acupuncture. *Int J Epidemiol* 2001 Jun; 30(3): 526–31.
33. Panzer, R. A comparison of the traditional Chinese vs. transpositional *zangfu* organ association acupoint locations in the horse. *Am J Chin Med* 1993; 21(2): 119–31.
34. Dung, H. C. Anatomical features which contribute to the formation of acupuncture points. *Am J Acupunct* 1984; 12: 139–44.
35. Langevin, H., Vaillancourt, P. Acupuncture: Does it work and, if so, how? *Sem Clin Neuropsych* 1999; 4(3): 167–75.
36. Cho, S-H., Chun, S. I. The basal electrical skin resistance of acupuncture points in normal subjects. *Yonsei Med J* 1994; 35: 464–73.
37. Noordergraaf, S., Silage, D. Electroacupuncture. *EEEE Trans Biomed Eng* 1973; 20: 364–66.
38. Hot, P., et al. Diurnal variations of tonic electrodermal activity. *Int J Psychophysiol* 1999; 33(3): 223–30.
39. Yamamoto, T., et al. Measurement of low-resistance points on the skin by dry roller electrodes. *IEEE Trans Biomed Eng* 1988; 35(3): 203–9.
40. Yamamoto, T., Yamamoto, Y. Analysis for the change of skin impedance. *Med Biol Eng Comput* 1977; 15(3): 219–27.
41. Coyle, M., et al. The *cun* measurement system: An investigation into its suitability in current practice. *Acupunct Med* 2000; 18(1): 10–14.
42. Aird, M., et al. A study of the comparative accuracy of two methods of locating acupuncture points. *Acupunct Med* 2000; 18(1): 15–21.
43. Aird, M., Cobbin, D. M., Rogers, C. A study of the relative precision of acupoint location methods. *J Altern Complement Med* 2002; 8(5): 635–42.
44. Mann, F., in Filshie, J., White, A. (eds.), *Medical acupuncture: A Western scientific approach.* London: Churchill Livingstone, 1998; 62.
45. Sanchez Aranjo, M. Does the choice of placebo determine the results of clinical studies on acupuncture? *Forsch Komplementarmed* 1998; 5 Suppl S1: 8–11

46. Panzer, R., op. cit.
47. Ernst, E. Complementary medicine: The facts. *Phys The Rev* 1997; 2: 49–57.
48. Ramey, D. W., Buell, P. B. Do acupuncture points and meridians actually exist? *Compendium on Continuing Education for the Practicing Veterinarian*, 2000; 22(12): 1132.
49. Hui, K. K., et al. Acupuncture modulates the limbic system and subcortical gray structures of the human brain: Evidence from fMRI studies in normal subjects. *Hum Brain Mapp* 2000; 9(1): 13–25.
50. Li, G., et al. An fMRI study comparing brain activation between word generation and electrical stimulation of language-implicated acupoints. *Hum Brain Mapp* 2003; 18(3): 233–38.
51. Vincent, C. A., et al. The significance of needle placement site in acupuncture. *J Psychosom Res* 1989; 33(4): 489–96.
52. Zaslawski, C. J., et al. The impact of site specificity and needle manipulation on changes to pain pressure threshold following manual acupuncture: A controlled study. *Complement Ther Med* 2003; 11(1): 11–21.
53. Suter, B., Kistler, A. [Demonstration of the effect of acupuncture on the autonomic nervous system by examination of the microcirculation]. *Forsch Komplementar Med* 1999 Feb; 6 Suppl 1: 32–34. [in German]
54. Iranmanesh, A., Lizarralde, G., Veldhuis, J. D. Coordinate activation of the corticotropic axis by insulin-induced hypoglycemia: Simultaneous estimates of beta-endorphin, adrenocorticotropin and cortisol secretion and disappearance in normal men. *Acta Endocrinol (Copenh)* 1993; 128(6): 521–28.
55. Max, M. B., et al. Epidural and intrathecal opiates: Cerebrospinal fluid and plasma profiles in patients with chronic cancer pain. *Clin Pharmacol Ther* 1985; 38(6): 631–41.
56. Skarda, R. T., Tejwani, G. A., Muir, W. W., 3rd. Cutaneous analgesia, hemodynamic and respiratory effects, and beta-endorphin concentration in spinal fluid and plasma of horses after acupuncture and electroacupuncture. *Am J Vet Res* 2002; 63(10): 1435–42.
57. Li, W. I., Chen, C. L. Running and shipping elevate plasma levels of beta-endorphin-like substance (B-END-LI) in thoroughbred horses. *Life Sci* 1987, Apr 6; 40(14): 1411–21.
58. ter Riet, G., et al. Is placebo analgesia mediated by endogenous opioids? A systematic review. *Pain* 1998 Jun; 76(3): 273–75.
59. Cheng, R. S. S., et al. Electroacupuncture elevates blood cortisol levels in naive horses; sham treatment has no effect. *Intl J Neuroscience* 1980; 10: 95–97.
60. Glardon, O. J. Variation of plasma cortisol values in horses after acupuncture. *Pratique Veterinaire Equine* 1988; 20: 32–34.

61. Kalauokalani, D., et al. Lessons from a trial of acupuncture and massage for low back pain: Patient expectations and treatment effects. *Spine* 2001, Jul 1; 26(13): 1418–24.

62. Levine, J. D., Gormley, J., Fields, H. L. Observations on the analgesic effects of needle puncture (acupuncture). *Pain.* 1976; 2(2): 149–59.

63. Bing, Z., Villanueva, L., Le Bars, D. Acupuncture and diffuse noxious inhibitory controls: Naloxone-reversible depression of activities of trigeminal convergent neurons. *Neuroscience* 1990; 37(3): 809–18.

64. Murase, K., Kawakita, K. Diffuse noxious inhibitory controls in anti-noci-ception produced by acupuncture and moxibustion on trigeminal cau-dalis neurons in rats. *Jpn J Physiol* 2000 Feb; 50(1): 133–40. In this study, pinch stimulation induced the most profound suppression followed by manual acupuncture. Moxibustion induced moderate suppression with a long induction time. These results suggest that diffuse noxious inhibitory controls may be involved in the analgesic mechanism of acupuncture and moxibustion.

65. Skarda, R. T., Muir, W. W. Comparison of electroacupuncture and butor-phanol on respiratory and cardiovascular effects and rectal pain thresh-old after controlled rectal distention in mares. *Am J Vet Res* 2003; 64(2): 137–44.

66. Rushton, D. N. Electrical stimulation in the treatment of pain. *Disabil Rehabil* 2002; 24(8): 407–15.

67. Ulett, G. A., Han, S., Han, J. S. Electroacupuncture: Mechanisms and clinical application. *Biol Psychiatry* 1998; 44(2): 129–38.

68. Alt-Epping, S., et al. [Diagnostics of appendicitis in a particular consider-ation of the acupunture point lanwei—a prospective study]. Forsch Komplementarmed Klass Naturheilkd, 2002; 9(6): 338–45 [in German].

69. Fenger, C. K., et al. Equine protozoal myelitis: Acupuncture diagnosis. *Proc 43rd Am Assn Equine Practitions* 1997; 327–29.

70. Sato, M., et al. Peroneal nerve palsy following acupuncture treatment: A case report. *J Bone Joint Surg Am* 2003; 85-A(5): 916–18.

71. Woo, P. C., et al. *Staphylococcus aureus* subcutaneous abscess complicat-ing acupuncture: Need for implementation of proper infection control guidelines. *New Microbiol* 2003; 26(2): 169–74.

72. Lao, L., et al. Is acupuncture safe? A systematic review of case reports. *Altern Ther Health Med* 2003; 9(1): 72–83.

73. MacPherson, H., et al. A prospective survey of adverse events and treat-ment reactions following 34,000 consultations with professional acupuncturists. *Acupunct Med* 2001 Dec; 19(2): 93–102.

74. Haldeman, S. Neurologic effects of the adjustment. *Journal of Manipula-tive & Physiological Therapeutics* 2000 (Feb); 23(2): 112–14.

75. Nelson, C. F. The subluxation question. *Journal of Chiropractic Humanities* 1997; 7: 46–55.
76. French, S. D., Green, S., Forbes, A. Reliability of chiropractic methods commonly used to detect manipulable lesions in patients with chronic low-back pain. *J Manipulative Physiol Ther* 2000; 23(4): 231–38.
77. Hestbaek, L., Leboeuf-Yde, C. Are chiropractic tests for the lumbo-pelvic spine reliable and valid? A systematic critical literature review. *J Manipulative Physiol Ther* 2000; 23(4): 258–75.
78. Shekelle, P. G., et al. *The appropriateness of spinal manipulation for low-back pain: Project overview and literature review.* Santa Monica, CA: RAND Corporation, 1991 (Document #R-4025/1-CCR/FCER).
79. Coulter, I. D., et al. *The appropriateness of manipulation and mobilization of the cervical spine.* Santa Monica, CA: RAND Corporation, 1996.
80. Shekelle, P. G., et al. Spinal manipulation for low back pain. *Ann Int Med* 1992; 117: 590–98.
81. Koes, B. W., et al. Spinal manipulation for low back pain. An updated systematic review of randomized clinical trials. *Spine* 1996; 21: 2860–71.
82. Hurwitz, E. L., et al. Manipulation and mobilization of the cervical spine. A systematic review of the literature. *Spine* 1996; 21: 1746–59.
83. Anderson, R., et al. A meta-analysis of clinical trials of spinal manipulation. *J Manip Physiol Ther* 1992; 15: 181–94.
84. Aker, P. D., et al. Conservative management of mechanical neck pain: Systematic review and meta-analysis. *BMJ* 1996; 313: 1291–96.
85. Assendelft, W. J., et al. The relationship between methodological quality and conclusions in reviews of spinal manipulation. *JAMA* 1995; 274: 1942–48.
86. Koes, B. W., et al. Randomised clinical trial of manipulative therapy and physiotherapy for persistent back and neck complaints: Results of one year follow up. *BMJ* 1992; 304(6827): 601–5.
87. Ernst, E., Harkness, E. Spinal manipulation: A systematic review of sham-controlled, double-blind, randomized clinical trials. *J Pain Symptom Manage.* 2001 Oct; 22(4): 879–89.
88. Cherkin, D. C., et al. A comparison of physical therapy, chiropractic manipulation, and provision of an educational booklet for the treatment of patients with low back pain. *N Engl J Med* 1998 Oct 8; 339(15): 1021–29.
89. Bronfort, G., Assendelft, W. J., Bouter, L. Efficacy of spinal manipulative therapies for conditions other than neck and back pain: A systematic review and best evidence synthesis. *Proc Int Conf on Spinal Manipulation*, 1996, Bournemouth, UK. Brookline, MA: Foundation for Chiropractic Education and Research; 1996: 105–6.

90. Hondras, M. A., Linde, K., Jones, A. P. Manual therapy for asthma. *Cochrane Database Systematic Review* 2001; I: CD0001001 [PMID: 11279701].

91. Cooper, R. A., McKee, H. J. Chiropractic in the United States: Trends and issues. *Milbank Q* 2003; 81(1): 107–38.

92. Assendelft, W. J., et al. Spinal manipulative therapy for low back pain. *Ann Intern Med* 2003; 138: 871–81.

93. Keating, J. C., et al. Inter-examiner reliability of eight evaluative dimensions of lumbar segmental abnormality. *Journal of Manipulative & Physiological Therapeutics* 1990, Oct; 13(8): 463–70.

94. Boline, P. D., et al. Interexaminer reliability of eight, evaluative dimensions of lumbar segmental abnormality: Part II. *Journal of Manipulative & Physiological Therapeutics* 1993 July/Aug; 16(6): 363–74.

95. Bergman, T. F., Peterson, D. H., Lawrence, D. J. *Chiropractic technique: Principles and procedures.* New York: Churchill Livingstone, 1993.

96. Cooperstein, R. Contemporary approach to understanding chiropractic technique. In Lawrence, D. J., et al., eds., *Advances in chiropractic*, vol. 2. St. Louis: Mosby-Year Book, 1995; 437–59.

97. Keating, J. C., Jr. Several pathways in the evolution of chiropractic manipulation. *J Manipulative Physiol Ther* 2003; 26(5): 300–21.

98. Hurwitz, E. L., et al. The effectiveness of physical modalities among patients with low back pain randomized to chiropractic care: Findings from the UCLA low back pain study. *J Manipulative Physiol Ther* 2002; 25(1): 10–20.

99. Keating, J. C. To hunt the subluxation: Clinical research considerations. *J Manipulative Physiol Ther* 1996; 19(9): 613–19.

100. Keating, J. C., Mootz, R. D. The influence of political medicine on chiropractic dogma: Implications for scientific development. *J Manipulative Physio Ther* 1989; 12(5): 393–98.

101. Keating, J. C., Green, B. N., Johnson, C. D. "Research" and "science" in the first half of the chiropractic century. *J Manipulative Physiol Ther* 1995; 18(6): 357–78.

102. More medicaid cuts loom for chiropractic (http: //www.chiroweb.com/archives/21/11/15.html; accessed April 29, 2003).

103. Grod, J. P., Sikorski, D., Keating, J. C., Jr. Unsubstantiated claims in patient brochures from the largest state, provincial, and national chiropractic associations and research agencies. *J Manipulative Physiol Ther* 2001; 24(8): 514–19.

104. Gatterman, M. I., ed. *Foundations of chiropractic: Subluxation.* St. Louis: Mosby, 1995.

105. Nansel, D. D., et al. Effect of unilateral spinal adjustments on goniometrically-assessed cervical lateral-flexion end-range asymmetries in otherwise asymptomatic subjects. *J Manip Physiol Ther* 1989; 12: 419–27.

106. Mierau, D. Manipulation and mobilization of the third metacarpopha-
langeal joint: A quantitative radiographic and range of motions study.
Manual Med 1988: 3: 135–40.

107. Cramer, G. D., et al. Effects of side-posture positioning and side-posture
adjusting on the lumbar zygapophysial joints as evaluated by MRI: A
before and after study with randomization. *J Manip Physiol Ther* 2000;
23: 380–94.

108. Terrett, A. C., Vernon, H. Manipulation and pain tolerance. A controlled study of the effect of spinal manipulation on paraspinal cutaneous pain tolerance levels. *Am J Phys Med* 1984; 63: 217–25.

109. Vernon, H. T., et al. Spinal manipulation and beta-endorphin: A
controlled study of the effect of a spinal manipulation of plasma beta-
endorphin levels in normal males. *J Manip Physiol Ther* 1986; 9:
115–23.

110. Crelin, E. S. A scientific test of the chiropractic theory. *Am Sci* 1973 Sep-
Oct; 61(5): 574–80. See also http://www.chirobase.org/02Research/
crelin.html.

111. Herzog, W., Kats, M., Symons, B. The effective forces transmitted by
high-speed, low-amplitude thoracic manipulation. *Spine* 2001 Oct 1;
26(19): 2105–10.

112. Shekelle, P. G., op. cit.

113. Smith, W. S., et al. Spinal manipulative therapy in an independent risk
factor for vertebral artery dissection. *Neurology* 2003; 60: 1424–28.

114. Haldeman, S., Kohlbeck, F. J., McGregor, M. Risk factors and precipitat-
ing neck movements causing vertebrobasilar artery dissection after cervical trauma and spinal manipulation. *Spine* 1999; 24: 785–94.

115. Hill, C., Doyon, F. Review of randomized trials of homeopathy. *Rev
Epidme et Sante Publ* 1990; 38: 139–47.

116. Kleijnen, J., Knipschild, P., ter Riet, G. Clinical trials of homeopathy.
BMJ 1991; 302: 316–23.

117. Kleijnen, J., Knipschild, P., ter Riet, G. Trials of homeopathy. *BMJ* 1991;
302: 960.

118. Kurz, R. [Clinical medicine versus homeopathy]. *Padiatr Padol* 1992;
27(2): 37–41 [in German].

119. Linde, K., et al. Critical review and meta-analysis of serial agitated dilutions in experimental toxicology. *Human & Exper Toxicol* 1994; 13:
481–92.

120. Aulas, J. Homeopathy update. *Préscrire International* 1996; 15(155): 674–84.

121. Linde, K., et al. Are the clinical effects of homeopathy placebo effects? A
meta-analysis of placebo-controlled trials. *Lancet* 1997; 350: 834–43.

122. Langman, M. J. S. Homeopathy trial: Reason for good ones but are they
warranted? *Lancet* 1997; 350: 825.

123. Vandenbroucke, J. P. Homeopathy trials: Going nowhere. *Lancet* 1997; 350: 824.

124. Linde, K., et al. Impact of study quality on outcome in placebo-controlled trials of homeopathy. *J Clin Epidemiol* 1999; 52(7): 631–36.

125. Barnes, J., Resch, K., Ernst, E. Homeopathy for post-operative ileus? A meta-analysis. *J Clin Gastro* 1997; 25(4): 628–33.

126. Vickers, A. J. Independent relication of preclinical research in home-opathy: a systematic review. *Forsch Komplementarmed* 1999; 6: 311–20.

127. Ernst, E. A systematic review of systematic reviews of homeopathy. *British Journal of Clinical Pharmacology* 2002; 54: 577–82.

128. Jonas, W. B., Kaptchuk, T. J., Linde, K. A critical overview of homeopathy. *Ann Intern Med* 2003; 138(5): 393–99.

129. Friese, K., Feuchter, U., Moeller, H. Homeopathic management of adenoid vegetations. Results of a prospective, randomized double-blind study. *HNO* 1997; 45: 618–24.

130. Hart, O., et al. Double-blind, placebo-controlled, randomized clinical trial of homoeopathic arnica C30 for pain and infection after total abdominal hysterectomy. *J R Soc Med* 1997 Feb; 90(2): 73–78.

131. Whitmarsh, T., Coleston-shields, D., Steiner, T. Double-blind randomized placebo-controlled study of homeopathic prophylaxis of migraine. *Cephalgia* 1997; 17: 600–604.

132. Wallach, H., et al. Classical homeopathic treatment of chronic headaches. *Cephalgia* 1997; 17: 119–26.

133. Stevinson, C., et al. Homeopathic arnica for prevention of pain and bruising: Randomized placebo-controlled trial in hand surgery. *J R Soc Med* 2003; 96(2): 60–65.

134. Bonne, O., et al. A randomized, double-blind, placebo-controlled study of classical homeopathy in generalized anxiety disorder. *J Clin Psychiatry* 2003; 64(3): 282–87.

135. Lewith, G. T., et al. Use of ultramolecular potencies of allergen to treat asthmatic people allergic to house dust mite: Double blind randomised controlled clinical trial. *BMJ* 2002; 324(7336): 520.

136. White, A., et al. Individualised homeopathy as an adjunct in the treatment of childhood asthma: A randomized placebo controlled trial. *Thorax* 2003; 58: 317–21.

137. Ullman, D. *Discovering homeopathy: Medicine for the 21st century*. Berkeley, CA: North Atlantic Books, 1991.

138. Roberts, A., et al. The power of nonspecific effects in healing: Implications for psychological and biological treatments. *Clin Psychol Rev* 1993; 13: 375–91.

139. Wallach, H. Does a highly diluted homeopathic drug act as a placebo in healthy volunteers? Experimental study of Belladonna 30C in a double

blind crossover design—a pilot study. *J Psychosomatic Res* 1993; 37(8): 851–60.

140. Vickers, A. J., van Haselen, R., Heger, M. Can homeopathically prepared mercury cause symptoms in healthy volunteers? A randomized, double-blind placebo-controlled trial. *J Altern Complement Med* 2001; 7(2): 141–48.

141. Goodyear, K., Lewith, G., Low, J. L. Randomized double-blind placebo-controlled trial of homoeopathic "proving" for Belladonna C30. *J R Soc Med* 1998; 91(11): 579–82.

142. Aberer, W., et al. Homeopathic preparations—severe adverse effects, unproven benefits. *Dermatologia* 1991; 182(4): 253.

143. Kerr, H., Yarborough, G. Pancreatitis following ingestion of a homeopathic preparation. *N Engl J Med* 1986 Jun 19; 314(25): 1642–43.

144. van Ulsen J., Stolz, E., van Joost, T. Chromate dermatitis from a homeopathic drug. *Contact Dermatitis* 1988 Jan; 18(1): 56–57.

145. Ernst, E. The attitude against immunisation within some branches of complementary medicine. *Eur J Pediatr* 1997; 156: 513–15.

146. Ernst, E., White, A. R. Homeopathy and immunisation. *Br J Gen Pract* 1995; 48: 629–30.

147. Sulfaro, F., Fasher B., Burgess, M. A. Homeopathic vaccination. What does it mean? *Med J Austr* 1994; 161: 305–7.

148. Rasky, E., et al. Arbeits und Lebensweise von homöpathisch tSätigen Ärztinnen und Ärtzen in Österreich. *Wein Med Wochenschr* 1994; 17: 419–24 [in German].

149. Fisher, P. Enough nonsense on immunisation. *Br Homeopath J* 1990; 79: 198–200.

150. Ernst, E. Science and anti-science in complementary medicine. *Br J Hosp Med* 1995; 54(7): 304–5.

151. Pray, S. A challenge to the credibility of homeopathy. *Am J Pain Man* 1992; 2: 63–71.

152. Hahnemann, S. *Organon of medicine*, 6th ed. Los Angeles: JP Tarcher, 1982.

153. English, P. The issue of immunization. *Br Homeopath J* 1992; 81: 161–63.

154. Carlson, T., Bergquist, L., Hellgren, U. Homeopatiska medol ger falsk säkerhet. *Lakartidningen* 1995; 92: 4467–68 [in Swedish].

155. Fisher, P. Enough nonsense on immunization. *Br Homeopath J* 1990; 79: 198–200.

156. Aulas, J. J., Bardelay, G. L'homéopathie vétérinaire, in L'homéopathie: Approche historique et critique et évaluation scientifique de ses fondement empiriques et de son efficacité thérapeutique. Paris: Roland Bettex Publ, 1985: 209–24 [in French].

157. Löscher, W. Homöopathie in der Veterinärmedizin: Kritische Über-
legungen aus der Sicht der Pharmakologie. In *Unkonventionelle medi-
zinische Verfahren*, Oepen, I., ed. Stuttgart: Gustav Fischer Verlag 1993;
273–302 [in German].

158. Wynn, S. G. Studies on use of homeopathy in animals. *JAVMA* 1998;
212(5): 719–24.

159. Scott, D. W., et al. Treatment of canine atopic dermatitis with a commercial homeopathic remedy: A single-blinded, placebo-controlled
study. *Can Vet J* 2002; 43(8): 601–3.

160. Klingenberg, et al. Evaluation of the effect of homeopathic treatment of
neonatal calf enteritis. *Svensk-Veterinartidning* 2001; 53, 733–36.

161. Pavlov, I. *Conditioned reflexes*. Oxford University Press, 1927.

162. Larson, L. J., Wynn, S., Schultz, R. D. A canine parvovirus nosode study
(abstr). In *Proceedings, 2nd Ann Midwest Holistic Vet Conf* 1996; 98–99.

163. Taylor, S. M., Mallon, T. R., Green, W. P. Efficacy of a homoeopathic
prophylaxis against experimental infection of calves by the bovine lung-
worm *Dictyocaulus viviparus*. *Vet Rec* 1989; 124(1): 15–17.

164. Appel, M. J. Forty years of canine vaccination. *Adv Vet Med* 1999; 41:
309–24.

165. Cairns, J., in *Accomplishments in cancer research in the United States*, Fort-
ner, J. G., Rhoads, J. E., eds. Philadelphia, PA: J.B. Lippincott, 1986, 86.

166. Huxtable, R. A brief history of pharmacology, therapeutics and scientific thought. *Proc West Pharmacol Soc* 1999; 42: 181–223.

167. Vickers, A., Zollman, C. E. ABC of complementary medicine: Herbal
medicine. *BMJ* 1999, 319: 1050–1053

168. Bodeker, G. C. Editorial. *J Altern Complement Med* 1996, 3: 323–26.

169. Steuer-Vogt, M. K., et al. The effect of an adjuvant mistletoe treatment
programme in resected head and neck cancer patients: A randomised
controlled clinical trial. *Eur J Cancer* 2001; 37(1): 23–31.

170. Linde, K., et al. Systematic reviews of complementary therapies—an
annotated bibliography. Part 2: Herbal medicine. *BMC Complement
Altern Med* 2001; 1(1): 5

171. Temple, R., Ellenberg, S. S. Placebo-controlled trials and active-control
trials in the evaluation of new treatments. Part 1: Ethical and scientific
issues. *Ann Intern Med* 2000; 133(6): 455–63.

172. Mrlianova, M., Tekel'ova, D., Felklova, M., Reinohl, V., Toth, J. The
influence of the harvest cut height on the quality of the herbal drugs
Melissae folium and Melissae herba. *Planta Med* 2002 Feb; 68(2):
178–80.

173. Gilroy, C. M., et al. Echinacea and truth in labeling. *Arch Intern Med*
2003; 163: 699–704.

174. Ames, B. N., Profet, M., Gold, L. S. Dietary pesticides (99.99 percent all
natural). *Proc Natl Acad Sci* 1990; 87: 7777–81.

175. From the Centers for Disease Control and Prevention. Hepatic toxicity possibly associated with kava-containing products—United States, Germany, and Switzerland, 1999–2002. *JAMA* 2003; 289(1): 36–7.

176. Williamson, E. M. Synergy and other interactions in phytomedicines. *Phytomedicine* 2001; 8(5): 401–9.

177. Huxtable, R. J., Luthy, J., Zweifel, U. Toxicity of comfrey-pepsin preparations. *N Engl J Med* 1986 Oct 23; 315(17): 1095.

178. Ridker, P. M., et al. Hepatic venocclusive disease associated with the consumption of pyrrolizidine-containing dietary supplements. *Gastroenterology* 1985 Apr; 88(4): 1050–54.

179. Ernst, E. Harmless herbs? A review of the recent literature. *Am J Med* 1998 Feb; 104(2): 170–78.

180. Essler, D. Cancer and herbs. *N Engl J Med* 2000; 342: 1742–43.

181. Ernst, E. Second thoughts about safety of St. John's wort. *Lancet* 1999, 354: 2014–15.

182. De Smet, P. A. G. M. Health risks of herbal remedies. *Drug Safety* 1995; 13: 8193.

183. Miller, L. G. Herbal medicine. Selected clinical considerations focusing on known or potential drug-herb interactions. *Arch Intern Med* 1998, 158: 2200–2211.

184. Fugh-Berman, A. Herb-drug interactions. *Lancet* 2000; 355: 134–38.

185. Ernst, E. Possible interactions between synthetic and herbal medicinal products. Part 1: A systematic review of the indirect evidence. *Perfusion* 2000; 13: 415.

186. Ernst, E. Possible interactions between synthetic and herbal medicinal products. Part 2: A systematic review of the direct evidence. *Perfusion* 2000; 13: 6070.

187. Vanherweghem, L. J. Misuse of herbal remedies: The case of an outbreak of terminal renal failure in Belgium (Chinese herbs nephropathy). *J Altern Complement Med* 1998 Spring; 4(1): 9–13.

188. Ko, R. J. Adulterants in Asian patent medicines. *N Engl J Med* 1998 Sep 17; 339(12): 847.

189. But, P. P. Herbal poisoning caused by adulterants or erroneous substitutes. *J Trop Med Hyg* 1994; 97(6): 371–74.

190. Chan, T. Y., et al. Chinese herbal medicines revisited: A Hong Kong perspective. *Lancet* 1993 Dec 18–25; 342 (8886–87): 1532–34.

191. Lau, K. K., Lai, C. K., Chan, A. W. Phenytoin poisoning after using Chinese proprietary medicines. *Hum Exp Toxicol* 2000 Jul; 19 (7): 385–86.

192. Sovak, M., et al. Herbal composition PC-SPES for management of prostate cancer: Identification of active principles. *J Natl Cancer Inst* 2002; 94(17): 1275–81.

193. Marcus, D. M., Grollman, A. P. Botanical medicines—the need for new regulations. *N Engl J Med* 2002; 347(25): 2073–76.

194. Means, C. Selected herbal hazards. *Vet Clin North Am Small Anim Pract* 2002 Mar; 32(2): 367–82.

195. Villar, D., Knight, M. J., Hansen, S. R. Toxicity of melaleuca oil and related essential oils applied topically on dogs and cats. *Vet Hum Toxicol* 1994; 36(2): 139–42.

196. Poppenga, R. H. Herbal medicine: Potential for intoxication and interactions with conventional drugs. *Clin Tech Small Anim Pract* 2002; 17(1): 6–18.

197. http://www.vbma.org/; accessed July 11, 2003.

198. Kellaway, P. The part played by electric fish in the early history of bioelectricity and electrotherapy. *Bull Hist Med* 1946; 20: 112–37.

199. Polk, C. Electric and magnetic fields for bone and soft tissue repair. In *Handbook of biological effects of electromagnetic fields*, 2nd ed., Polk, C. and Postow, E., eds. Boca Raton, FL: CRC Press, 1996; 231–46.

200. Schulten, K. Magnetic field effects in chemistry and biology. *Adv Solid State Phys* 22: 61, 1982.

201. Steiner, U. E., Ulrich, T. Magnetic field effects in chemical kinetics and related phenomena. *Chem Rev* 1989; 89: 51.

202. Beall, P. T., Hazlewood, C. F., Rao, P. N. Nuclear magnetic resonance patterns of intracellular water as a function of HeLa cell cycle. *Science* 1976; 192: 904–7.

203. Frankel, R. B., Liburdy, R. P. Biological effects of static magnetic fields. In Polk, C., Postow, E. *Handbook of biological effects of electromagnetic fields*, 2nd ed. Boca Raton, FL: CRC Press, 1996; 149–83.

204. Ishisaka, R., et al. Effects of a magnetic field on the various functions of subcellular organelles and cells. *Pathophysiology* 2000; 7(2): 149–52.

205. Blechman, A. M., et al. Discrepancy between claimed field flux density of some commercially available magnets and actual gaussmeter measurements. *Altern Ther Health Med* 2001; 7(5): 92–95.

206. Davidovitch, Z., et al. Biochemical mediators of the effects of mechanical forces in electric currents on mineralized tissue. *Calcif Tissue Int* 1984; 36 (Suppl 1): 586–597.

207. Aaron, R., Ciombor, D. Acceleration of experimental endochondral ossification by biophysical stimulation of the progenitor cell pool. *J Orthop Res* 1996; 14(4): 582–89.

208. Cho, M., et al. Reorganization of microfilament structure induced by ac electric fields. *FASEB J* 1996; 10: 1552–58.

209. MacGinitie, L. A., Gluzbank, Y. A., Grodzinski, A. J. Electric field stimulation can increase protein synthesis in articular cartilage explants. *J Orthop Res* 1994; 12: 151–60.

210. Saygili, G., et al. Investigation of the effect of magnetic retention systems used in prosthodontics on buccal mucosal blood flow. *Int J of Prosthodont* 1992; 5(4): 326–32.

211. Belossi, A., et al. No effect of a low-frequency pulsed magnetic field on the brain blood flow among mice. *Panminerva Med* 1993; 35(1): 57–59.

212. Barker, A., Cain, M. The claimed vasodilatory effect of a commercial permanent magnet foil; results of a double blind trial. *Clin Phys Physiol Meas* 1985; 6(3): 261–63.

213. Mayrovitz, H. N., et al. Effects of permanent magnets on resting skin blood perfusion in healthy persons assessed by laser Doppler flowmetry and imaging. *Bioelectromagnetics* 2001; 22(7): 494–502.

214. Turner, T., Wolfsdorf, K., Jourdenais, J. Effects of heat, cold, biomagnets and ultrasound on skin circulation in the horse. *Proc 37th AAEP* 1991; 249–57.

215. Steyn, P. F., et al. Effect of a static magnetic field on blood flow to the metacarpus in horses. *J Am Vet Med Assoc* 2000; 217(6): 874–77.

216. Stick, C., et al. Do Strong magnetic fields in NMR tomography modify tissue perfusion? *Nuklearmedizin* 1991; 154: 326.

217. Keltner, J., et al. Magnetohydrodynamics of blood flow. *Mag Res in Med* 1990; 16: 139.

218. Shimizu, T., et al. Bone ingrowth into porous calcium phosphate ceramics; influence of pulsating electromagnetic field. *J Orthop Res* 1988; 6: 248–58.

219. Rubin, C., McLeod, K., Lanyon, L. Prevention of osteoporosis by pulsed electromagnetic fields. *J Bone Joint Surg [Am]* 1989; 71: 411–16.

220. Cruess, R., Bassett, C. A. L. The effect of pulsing electromagnetic fields on bone metabolism in experimental disuse osteoporosis. *Clin Orthop* 1983; 173: 345–50.

221. Miller, G., et al. Electromagnetic stimulation of canine bone grafts. *J Bone and Joint Surg [Am]* 1984; 66: 693–98.

222. Kold, S., Hickman, J. Preliminary study of quantitative aspects and the effect of pulsed electromagnetic field treatment on the incorporation of equine cancellous bone grafts. *Eq Vet J* 1987; 19(2): 120–24.

223. Sharrard, W. A double blind trial of pulsed electromagnetic fields for delayed union of tibial fractures. *J Bone and Joint Surg [Br]* 1990; 72: 347–55.

224. De Haas, W. G., Lazarovici, M. A., Morrison, D. M. The effect of low frequency magnetic field on healing of osteotomized rabbit radius. *Clin Orthop* 1979; 145: 245–51.

225. Leisner, S., et al. The effect of short-duration, high-intensity electromagnetic pulses on fresh ulnar fractures in rats. *J Vet Med A Physiol Pathol Clin Med* 2002; 49(1): 33–37.

226. Barker, A. T. Pulsating electromagnetic field therapy for the treatment of tibial non-union fractures. *Lancet* 1984; 8384 (1): 994–96.

227. Ieran, M., et al. Effect of low frequency pulsing electromagnetic fields on skin ulcers of venous origin in humans: A double-blind study. *J Orthop Res* 1990; 8(2): 276–82.

228. Kort, J., Ito, H., Basset, C. A. L. Effects of pulsing electromagnetic fields on peripheral nerve regeneration. *J Bone Jt Sug Orthop Trans* 1980; 4: 238.

229. Sisken, B. F., et al. Pulsed electromagnetic fields stimulate nerve regeneration in vitro and in vivo. *Restorative neurology and neuroscience* 1990b; 1: 303–309.

230. Polk, C. Electric and magnetic fields for bone and soft tissue repair. In *Handbook of biological effects of electromagnetic fields*, 2nd ed. Polk, C., Postow, E., eds. Boca Raton, FL: CRC Press, 1996, 231–46.

231. Bassett, C. A. L. Beneficial effects of electromagnetic fields. *J of Cell Biochem* 1993; 51: 387–93.

232. Lee, E. W., et al. Pulsed magnetic and electromagnetic fields in experimental Achilles tendonitis in the rat: A prospective randomized study. *Arch Phys Med and Rehab* 1997; 78(4): 399–404.

233. Robotti, E., et al. The effect of pulsed electromagnetic fields on flexor tendon healing in chickens. *J Hand Surg [Br]*. 1999; 24(1): 56–58.

234. Barker, A. T. Electricity, magnetism and the body: Some uses and abuses. *Eng Sci and Edu J*, 1993, Dec; 249–56.

235. Wikswo, J. P., Barach, J. P. An estimate of the steady magnetic field strength required to influence nerve conduction. *IEEE Transactions on Biomedical Engineering BME* 1980; 27(12): 722–23.

236. Lin, V. W., Hsiao, I., Kingery, W. S. High intensity magnetic stimulation over the lumbosacral spine evokes antinociception in rats. *Clin Neurophysiol* 2002; 113(7): 1006–12.

237. Trock, D. H., Bollet, A. J., Markill, R. The effect of pulsed electromagnetic fields in the treatment of osteoarthritis of the knee and cervical spine. Report of randomized, double blind, placebo controlled trials. *J Rheumatol* 1994; 21(10): 1903–11.

238. Trock, D. H., et al. A double-blind trial of the clinical effects of pulsed electromagnetic fields in osteoarthritis. *J Rheumatol* 1993; 20(3): 456–60.

239. Foley-Nolan, D., et al. Pulsed high frequency (27MHz) electromagnetic therapy for persistent neck pain: A double blind, placebo-controlled study of 20 patients. *Orthopedics* 1990; 13(4): 445–51.

240. Varcaccia-Garofalo, G., et al. Analgesic properties of electromagnetic field therapy in patients with chronic pelvic pain. *Clin Exp Obstet Gynecol* 1995; 22(4): 350–54.

241. Leclaire, R., Bourgouin, J. Electromagnetic treatment of shoulder periarthritis: A randomized controlled trial of the efficiency and tolerance of magnetotherapy. *Arch Phys Med Rehabil* 1991; 72(5): 284–87.

242. Puett, D. W., Griffin, M. R. Published trials of nonmedicinal and noninvasive therapies for hip and knee osteoarthritis. *Ann Intern Med* 1994; 121(2): 133–40.

243. Papi, F., et al. Exposure to oscillating magnetic fields influences sensitivity to electrical stimuli, II. Experiments on humans. *Bioelectromagnetics* 1995; 16: 295–300.

244. Nakagawa, K. Clinical application of magnetic field. *J Soc Non-trad. Technol* 1974; 66: 6–17.

245. Nakagawa, K. Magnetic field-deficient syndrome and magnetic treatment. *Jap Med J* 1976; 2745: 24–32.

246. Vallbonna, C., Hazlewood, C. F., Jurida, G. Response of pain to static magnetic fields in postpolio patients: A double-blind pilot study. *Arch Phys Med Rehabil* 1997; 78: 1200–1204.

247. Weintraub, M. Magnetic biostimulation in painful diabetic peripheral neuropathy: A novel intervention—a randomized, double-placebo crossover study. *Am J Pain Manage* 1999; 9: 8–17.

248. Weintraub, M. I., et al. Static magnetic field therapy for symptomatic diabetic neuropathy: a randomized, double-blind, placebo-controlled trial. Arch Phys Med Rehabil 2003; 84(5): 736-46.

249. Hinman, M. R., Ford, J., Heyl, H. Effects of static magnets on chronic knee pain and physical function: A double-blind study. *Altern Ther Health Med* 2002; 8(4): 50–55.

250. Casselli, M. A., et al. Evaluation of magnetic foil and PPT Insoles in the treatment of heel pain. *J Am Podiatr Med Assoc* 1997; 87(1): 11–16.

251. Hong, C., et al. Magnetic necklace: Its therapeutic effectiveness on neck and shoulder pain. *Arch Phys Med Rehab* 1982; 63: 464–66.

252. Caselli, M. A., et al. Evaluation of magnetic foil and PPT insoles in the treatment of heel pain. *J Am Podiatr Med Assoc.* 1997; 87(1): 11–16.

253. Collacott, E. A., et al. Bipolar permanent magnets for the treatment of chronic low back pain. A pilot study. *JAMA* 2000; 283: 1322–25.

254. *Consumer Reports*, May 2000.

255. Lin, J. C., et al. Geophysical variables and behavior: XXVII. Magnetic necklace: Its therapeutic effectiveness on neck and shoulder pain: 2. Psychological assessment. *Psychological Reports* 1985; 56: 639–49.

256. Watkins, J., et al. Healing of surgically created defects in the equine superficial digital flexor tendon: Effects of PEMF on collagen-type transformation and tissue morphologic reorganization. *Am J Vet Res* 1985; 46: 2097–2103.

257. Bramlage, L., Weisbrode, S., Spurlock, G. The effect of a pulsating electromagnetic field on the acute healing of equine cortical bone. *Proc 30th AAEP* 1984; 43–48.

258. Cane, V., Botti, P., Soana, S. Pulsed magnetic fields improve osteoblast activity during the repair of an experimental osseous defect. *J Ortho Research* 1993; 11(5): 664–70.

259. Collier, M., et al. Radioisotope uptake in normal equine bone under the influence of a pulsed electromagnetic field. *Mod Vet Prac* 1985; 66: 971–74.

260. Jauchem, J. R., Merritt, J. H. The epidemiology of exposure to electromagnetic fields: An overview of the recent literature. *J Clin Epidemiol* 1991; 44: 895–906.

261. Michaelson, S. M. Influence of power frequency electric and magnetic fields on human health. *Ann N Y Acad Sci* 1987; 502: 55–75.

262. Shore, R. E. Electromagnetic radiations and cancer. Cause and prevention. *Cancer* 1988; 62: 1747–54.

263. Kaiser, J. Panel finds EMFs pose no threat [news] [see comments] [published erratum appears in *Science* 1997 Feb 7; 275(5301): 741]. *Science* 1996; 274: 910.

264. Philadelphia panel evidence-based clinical practice guidelines on selected rehabilitation interventions for knee pain. *Phys Ther* 2001; 81(10): 1675–99.

265. Philadelphia panel evidence-based clinical practice guidelines on selected rehabilitation interventions for low back pain. *Phys Ther* 2001; 81(10): 1701–17.

266. Ulett, G. A., Han, S., Han, J. S. Electroacupuncture: Mechanisms and clinical application. *Biol Psychiatry* 1998; 44(2): 129–38.

267. Ulett, G. A., Han, J., Han, S. Traditional and evidence-based acupuncture: History, mechanisms, and present status. *South Med J* 1998; 91(12): 1115–20.

268. Corazza, M., et al. Accelerated allergic contact dermatitis to a transcutaneous electrical nerve stimulation device. *Dermatology* 1999; 199(3): 281.

269. Stefanatos, J. Introduction to bioenergetic medicine. In *Complementary and alternative veterinary medicine: Principles and practice*, Schoen, A., Wynn, S., eds. St. Louis, MO: Mosby, 1997.

270. McDonagh, A. F. Phototherapy: From ancient Egypt to the new millenium. *J Perinatology* 2001; 21: S7–S12.

271. Enwemeka, C. S. Ultrastructural morphometry of membrane-bound intracytoplasmic collagen fibrils in tendon fibroblasts exposed to He:Ne laser beam. *Tissue Cell* 1992; 24: 511–23.

272. Basford, J. R. Low intensity laser therapy: Still not an established clinical tool. *Lasers Surg Med* 1995; 16: 331–42.

273. Kolari, P. J. Penetration of unfocused laser light into the skin. *Arch Dermatol Res* 1985; 277: 342–44.

274. Vizi, E. S., et al. Acetylcholine releasing effect of laser irradiation on Auerbach's plexus in guinea pig ileum. *J Neural Transm Park Dis Dement Sect* 1977; 40: 305.

275. Greathouse, D. G., Currier, D. P., Gilmore, R. L. Effects of clinical infrared laser on superficial radial nerve conduction. *Phys Ther* 1985; 65: 1184.

276. Enwemeka, C. S. Ultrastructural morphometry of membrane-bound intracytoplasmic collagen fibrils in tendon fibroblasts exposed to He:Ne laser beam. *Tissue Cell* 1992; 24: 511–23.

277. Karu, T. I. Photobiological fundamentals of low-power laser therapy. *IEEE Journal of Quantum Electronics* 1987; QE-23: 1703.

278. Sato, H., et al. The effects of laser light on sperm motility and velocity in vitro. *Andrologia* 1984; 16: 23.

279. Passarella, S., et al. Increase of proton electrochemical potential and ATP synthesis in rat liver mitochondria irradiated in vitro by helium-neon laser. *FEBS Lett* 1984; 175: 95.

280. Fork, R. L. Laser stimulation of nerve cells in aphysia. *Science* 1971; 171: 907–8.

281. Young, S., et al. Macrophage responsiveness to light therapy. *Lasers Surg Med* 1989; 9: 497–505.

282. Mester, E., et al. Effect of laser rays on wound healing. *Am J Surg* 1971; 122: 532.

283. Lundeberg, T., Malm, M. Low-power HeNe laser treatment of venous leg ulcers. *Ann Plast Surg* 1991; 27: 537–39.

284. Santoianni, P., et al. Inadequate effect of helium-neon laser on venous leg ulcers. *Photodermatology* 1984; 1: 245–49.

285. Malm, M., Lundeberg, T. Effect of low power gallium arsenide laser on healing of venous ulcers. *Scan J Plast Reconstr Surg Hand Surg* 1991; 25(3): 249–51.

286. Lucas, C., et al. Wound healing in cell studies and animal model experiments by low level laser therapy; were clinical studies justified? a systematic review. *Lasers Med Sci* 2002; 17(2): 110–34.

287. England, S., et al. Low power laser therapy of shoulder tendonitis. *Scand J Rheum* 1989; 18: 427–31.

288. Vecchio, P., et al. A double-blind study of the effectiveness of low level laser treatment of rotator cuff tendinitis. *Br J Rheum* 1993; 32: 740–42.

289. Siebert, W., et al. What is the efficacy of "soft" and "mid" lasers in therapy of tendinopathies? A double-blind study. *Arch Orthop Truam Surg* 1987; 106(6): 358–63.

290. McLauchlan, G. J., Handoll, H. H. Interventions for treating acute and chronic Achilles tendinitis. *Cochrane Database Syst Rev* 2001; (2): CD000232.

291. Colov, H. C., et al. Convincing clinical improvement of rheumatoid arthritis by soft laser therapy (abstract). *Lasers Surg Med* 1987; 7: 77.
292. Heussler, J. K., et al. A double-blind randomised trial of low power laser treatment in rheumatoid arthritis. *Ann Rheum Dis* 1993; 52(10): 703–6.
293. Zvereva, K. V., Grunina, E. A. [The negative effects of low-intensity laser therapy in rheumatoid arthritis]. *Ter Arkh* 1996; 68(5): 22–24 [in Russian].
294. Bertolucci, L. E., Grey, T. Clinical comparative study of microcurrent electrical stimluation to mid-laser and placebo treatment in degenerative joint disease of the temporomandibular joint. *Cranio* 1995; 13(2): 116–20.
295. Stelian, J., et al. Improvement of pain and disability in elderly patients with degenerative osteoarthritis of the knee treated with narrow-band light therapy. *J Am Geriatr Soc* 1992; 40(1): 23–26.
296. Bulow, P. M., Jensen, H., Danneskiold-Samsoe, B. Low power Ga-Al-As laser treatment of painful osteoarthritis of the knee. A double-blind placebo-controlled study. *Scand J Rehabil Med* 1994; 26(3): 155–59.
297. Basford, J. R., et al. Low-energy helium neon laser treatment of thumb osteoarthritis. *Arch Phys Med Rehabil* 1987; 68(11): 794–97.
298. Axelsen, S. M., Bjerno, T. [Laser therapy of ankle sprain]. *Ugeskr Laeger* 1993; 155(48): 3908–11 [in Danish].
299. Brosseau, L., et al. Low level laser therapy for osteoarthritis and rheumatoid arthritis: A meta-analysis. *J Rheumatol* 2000; 27(8): 1961–69.
300. Roynesdal, A. K., et al. The effect of soft-laser application on postoperative pain and swelling. A double-blind, crossover study. *Int J Maxillofac Surg* 1993; 22(4): 242–45.
301. Gerschman, J. A., Ruben, J., Gebart-Eaglemont, J. Low level laser therapy for dentinal tooth hypersensitivity. *Aust Dent J* 1994; 39(6): 353–57.
302. Klein, R. G., Eek, B. C. Low-energy laser treatment and exercise for chronic low back pain: Double-blind controlled trial. *Arch Phys Med Rehabil* 1990; 71(1): 34–47.
303. Krasheninnikoff, M., et al. No effect of low power laser therapy in lateral epicondylitis. *Scand J Rheumatol* 1994; 23(5): 260–63.
304. Lowe, A. S., et al. Failure to demonstrate any hypoalgesic effect of low intensity laser irradiation (830nm) of Erb's point upon experimental ischaemic pain in humans. *Lasers Surg Med* 1997; 20(1): 69–76.
305. Roynesdal, A. K., et al. The effect of soft-laser application on postoperative pain and swelling. A double-blind, crossover study. *Int J Maxillofac Surg* 1993; 22(4): 242–45.
306. Olavi, A., et al. Effects of the infrared laser therapy at treated and non-treated trigger points. *Acupunct Electrother Res* 1989; 14(1): 9–14.

307. Thorsen, H., et al. Low level laser therapy for myofascial pain in the neck and shoulder girdle. A double-blind, cross-over study. *Scand J Rheumatol* 1992; 21(3): 139–41.

308. Ter Riet, G., Van Houtem, H., Knipschild, P. Health-care professionals' views of the effectiveness of pressure ulcer treatments. *Clin Exp Dermatol* 1992; 17: 328–31.

309. Rush, P. J., Shore, A. Physician perceptions of the value of physical modalities in the treatment of musculoskeletal disease. *Br J Rheumatol* 1994; 33: 566–68.

310. Bouter, L. M. [Insufficient scientific evidence for efficacy of widely used electrotherapy, laser therapy, and ultrasound treatment in physiotherapy] *Ned Tijdschr Geneeskd* 2000; 144(11): 502–5.

311. Beckerman, H., et al. The efficacy of laser therapy for musculoskeletal and skin disorders: A criteria-based meta-analysis of randomized clinical trials. *Phys Ther* 1992; 72(7): 483–91.

312. Gam, A. N., Thorsen, H., Lonnberg, F. The effect of low-level laser therapy on musculoskeletal pain: A meta-analysis. *Pain* 1993; 52(1): 63–66.

313. Ernst, E., Fialka, V. [Low-dose laser therapy: Critical analysis of clinical effect]. *Schweiz Med Wochenschr* 1993; 123(18): 949–54 [in German].

314. Puett, D. W., Griffin, M. R. Published trials of nonmedicinal and noninvasive therapies for hip and knee osteoarthritis. *Ann Intern Med* 1994; 121(2): 133–40.

315. Gross, A. R., et al. Conservative management of mechanical neck disorders. A systematic overview and meta-analysis. *Online J Curr Clin Trials* DOC NO 200–201 Jul 30, 1996.

316. Low-power lasers in medicine. A report by the Australian Health Technology Advisory Committee (AHTAC) June 1994. *Aust J Sci Med Sport* 1994; 26(3–4): 73–76.

317. Brockhaus, A., Elger, C. E. Hypalgesic efficacy of acupuncture on experimental pain in man. Comparison of laser acupuncture and needle acupuncture. *Pain* 1990; 43: 181–85.

318. Basford, J. R. Low intensity laser therapy: Still not an established clinical tool. *Lasers Surg Med* 1995; 16: 331–42.

319. Medrado, A. R., et al. Influence of low level laser therapy on wound healing and its biological action upon myofibroblasts. *Lasers Surg Med* 2003; 32(3): 239–44.

320. Quickenden, T. I., Daniels, L. L. Attempted biostimulation of division in *saccharomyces cerevisiae* using red coherent light. *Photochem Photobiol* 1993; 57: 272–78.

321. Colver, G. B., Priestly, G. C. Failure of a helium-neon laser to affect components of wound healing in vitro. *Br J Dermatol* 1989 Aug; 121(2): 179–86.

322. Yu, W., Naim, J. O., Lanzafame, R. J. Effects of photostimulation on wound healing in diabetic mice. *Lasers Surg Med* 1997; 20(1): 56–63.

323. Ghamsari, S. M., et al. Evaluation of low level laser therapy on primary healing of experimentally induced full thickness teat wounds in dairy cattle. *Vet Surg* 1997; 26(2): 114–20.

324. Kami, T., et al. Effects of low-power diode lasers on flap survival. *Ann Plast Surg* 1985; 14(3): 278–83.

325. Medrado, A. R., et al. Influence of low level laser therapy on wound healing and its biological action upon myofibroblasts. *Lasers Surg Med* 2003; 32(3): 239–44.

326. Braverman, B., et al. Effect of helium-neon and infrared laser irradiation on wound healing in rabbits. *Lasers Surg Med* 1989; 9(1): 50–58.

327. Surinchak, J. S., et al. Effects of low-level energy lasers on the healing of full-thickness skin defects. *Lasers Surg Med* 1983; 2(3): 267–74.

328. Becker, J. [Biostimulation of wound healing in rats by combined soft and middle power lasers]. *Biomed Tech (Berl)* 1990; 35(5): 98–101 [in German].

329. Hutschenreiter, G., et al. [Wound healing after laser and red light irradiation]. *Z Exp Chir* 1980; 13(2): 75–85 [in German].

330. McCaughan, J. S., Jr., et al. Effect of low-dose argon irradiation on rate of wound closure. *Lasers Surg Med* 1985; 5(6): 607–14.

331. Basford, J. R., et al. Comparison of cold-quartz ultraviolet, low-energy laser and occulasion in wound healing in a swine model. *Arch Phys Med Rehabil* 1986; 67(3): 151–54.

332. In de Braekt, M. M., et al. Effect of low level laser therapy on wound healing after palatal surgery in beagle dogs. *Lasers Surg Med* 1991; 11(5): 462–70.

333. Peterson, S. L., et al. The effect of low level laser therapy (LLLT) on wound healing in horses. *Equine Vet J* 1999; 31(3): 228–31.

334. Kaneps, A. J., et al. Laser therapy in the horse: Histopathologic response. *Am J Vet Res* 1984; 45(3): 581–82.

335. McKibbin, L. S., Paraschak, D. M. A study of the effects of lasering on chronic bowed tendons at Wheatley Hall Farm Limited, Canada, January, 1983. *Lasers Surg Med* 1983; 3(1): 55–59.

336. Marr, C. M., et al. Factors affecting the clinical outcome of injuries to the superficial digital flexor tendon in National Hunt and point-to-point racehorses. *Vet Rec* 1993; 132: 476–79.

337. Gomez-Villamandos, R. J., et al. He-Ne laser therapy by fibroendoscopy in the mucosa of the equine upper airway. *Lasers Surg Med* 1995; 16(2): 184–88.

338. McKibbin, L. S., Paraschak, D. Use of laser light to treat certain lesions in standardbreds. *Mod Vet Pract* 1983; 65(3): 210–13.

339. Martin, B. B., Jr., Klide, A. M. Treatment of chronic back pain in horses. Stimulation of acupuncture points with a low powered infrared laser. *Vet Surg* 1987; 16(1): 106–10.
340. Klide, A. M., Martin, B. B., Jr. Methods of stimulating acupuncture points for treatment of chronic back pain in horses. *J Am Vet Med Assoc* 1989; 195(10): 1375–79.
341. http://www.therapy.com/Welcome.htm; accessed July 4, 2003.
342. Jarvis, D., MacIver, B. M., Tanelian, D. L. Effects of He-Ne laser irradiation on corneal A-Delta and C-fiber nociceptor electrophysiology. Poster 105, S209, Supplement 5, Department of Anesthesia, Stanford University Medical Center, Stanford, CA, 94305, 1990 (SPON: m.Lo).
343. Dasgupta, A. Review of abnormal laboratory test results and toxic effects due to use of herbal medicines. *Am J Clin Pathol,* 2003; 120(1): 127–137.

Chapter 8

1. Ober, K. P. The pre-Flexnerian reports—Mark Twain's criticism of medicine in the United States. *Annals of Internal Medicine* 1997 Jan 15; 126: 157–63.
2. Twain, M. Official physic. In *Mark Twain: Collected tales, sketches, speeches, and essays, 1852–1890,* Budd, L. J., ed. New York: The Library of America, 1992; 228–30.
3. See especially P. K. Feyerabend, *Against method: Outline of an anarchistic theory of knowledge* (London: NLB, 1975); and *Science in a free society* (London: NLB, 1978).

Chapter 9

1. Robinson, M. Accidental genius. *Wired Magazine* 10(1): 2002 (http://www.wired.com/wired/archive/10.01/accidental.html; accessed November 14, 2002).
2. *Author's Note:* One might reasonably contest whether or not prayer is a form of alternative medicine.
3. Ni, H., Simile, C., Hardy, A. M. Utilization of complementary and alternative medicine by United States adults: Results from the 1999 national health interview survey. *Med Care* 2002 Apr; 40(4): 353–58.
4. Schoen, A. M. Results of a survey on educational and research programs in complementary and alternative veterinary medicine at veterinary medical schools in the United States. *JAVMA* 2000; 216(4): 502–9.
5. Survey of pet owners, 1999–2000. Lakewood, CO: American Animal Hospital Association, 2000.
6. Ulett, G. Acupuncture legislation: What is the point? *Sci Rev Alt Med* 2001; 5(4): 229–32.

7. Meeker, W. C., Haldeman, S. Chiropractic: A profession at the crossroads of mainstream and alternative medicine. *Ann Int Med* 2002; 136(3): 216–27.

8. Ang-Lee, M. K., Moss, J., Yuan, C. Herbal medicines and perioperative care. *JAMA* 2001; 286: 44–48.

9. Kessler D. Cancer and herbs. *N Engl J Med* 2000; 342: 1742–43.

10. For example, see MO Rev. Stat. § 340.200(24), KA Stat. Ann. § 47-816(g)(1), AL Code § 34-29-61(14), KY Rev. Stat. § 321.181(5), ME Rev. Stat. Ann. § 4853(7)(A), AR Code Ann. § 17-101-102(2)(A), among many others.

11. For example, see ID Code § 54-2103(26), Louisiana Admin. Code, Vol. 3, Title 45, Part LXXXXV, § 712: *Alternative Medicine.*

12. OK S.B. 1344 (1999).

13. See *Notice of Approval of Regulatory Action* (Gov. Code, Sec. 11349.3), OAL File no. 98-0401-01 S (May 6, 1998).

14. For example, see NE Stat. § 638.070.2(h).

15. Texas Admin. Reg. § 573.12–573.16.

16. For example, Kansas, defining chiropractic care as involving treatment of humans, Kan. Stat. Ann. § 65-2802(a) and Kan. Stat. Ann. § 65-2871.

17. 1994 MD Laws ch. 620.

18. See 80 Maryland Attorney General Opinion No. 95-401 (September 26, 1995), 1995 *Westlaw* 591319. See also *A.V.M.L.A. Newsletter* 1996 Apr; 1(3).

19. MD Code Ann. § 2-301(f)(12) (1997).

20. *Department of Consumer & Industry Services v. Hoffmann* (Mich. App. no. 201322, June 5, 1998). See also *A.V.M.L.A. Newsletter* 1998 Sept; 3(4).

21. Maurer, E. L. The animal chiropractic issue. *J Am Chiro Assn* 2000 (June): 44–49.

22. http://www.orthopt.org/committees_sigs/animal_pt_sig/; accessed May 24, 2002.

23. Connecticut Legislature, Proposed Bill No. 5209, LCO No. 864, 2003.

24. http://www.minutuscourses.com/courses.htm; accessed July 4, 2003.

25. Long, L., Huntley, A., Ernst, E. Which complementary and alternative therapies benefit which conditions? A survey of the opinions of 223 professional organizations. *Complement Ther Med* 2001; 9(3): 178–85.

26. Clinical practice guidelines in complementary and alternative medicine. An analysis of opportunities and obstacles. Practice and Policy Guidelines Panel, National Institutes of Health Office of Alternative Medicine. *Arch Fam Med* 1997; 6(2): 148–54.

27. Modern drugs, surgery and diagnostics: Select the best. Stay current on the latest advancements. http://www.ahvma.org/; accessed May 5, 2002.

28. http://www.altvetmed.com/intro.html. Accessed March 15, 2003.

29. Zollman, C., Vickers, A. What is complementary medicine. *BMJ* 1999; 693–96.
30. *Ralston v. Texas State Board of Veterinary Medical Examiners* (Travis County, Texas, No. 97-00203).
31. Article XVI, Sec. 31 of the Texas Constitution (1876) specifically states "no preference shall be given by law to any schools (systems) of medicine."
32. Keating, J. C. *BJ of Davenport: The early years of chiropractic.* Davenport, IA: Association for the History of Chiropractic, 1997; 58–64.
33. Dawes, R. M., Faust, D., Meehl, P. E. Statistical prediction versus clinical prediction: Improving what works. In *Handbook for data analysis in the behavioral sciences: Methodological issues,* Keren, G., Lewis, C., eds. Hillsdale, NJ: Erlbaum, 1993: 351–67.
34. Dawes, R. M., Faust, D., Meehl, P. E. Clinical judgment versus actuarial judgment. *Science* 1989; 243: 1668–74.
35. Rollin, B. An ethicist's commentary on the case of a veterinarian utilizing homeopathic therapy. *Can Vet J* 1995; 36: 268–69.
36. Eisenberg, D. M. Advising patients who seek alternative medical therapies. *Ann Intern Med* 1997; 127: 61–69.

Afterword

1. Henney, J. E. Statement by Jane E. Henney, M.D., Commissioner, Food and Drug Administration, Department of Health and Human Services before the Committee on Government Reform, U.S. House of Representatives, March 25, 1999 (http://www.fda.gov:80/ola/dietary.html).
2. Imrie, R., Ramey, D. The evidence for evidence based medicine. *Comp Ther Med* 2000; 8: 123–26.
3. Nichols, J. B. Medical sectarianism. *J Am Med Assn* 60(5): 331–37.

Appendix

1. Model Veterinary Practice Act. In *2001 AVMA membership directory and resource manual.* Schaumburg, IL: American Veterinary Medical Association, 2001; 319.

Index